AN INTRODUCTION TO NUCLEAR PHYSICS, WITH APPLICATIONS IN MEDICINE AND BIOLOGY

N. A. DYSON, M.A., Ph.D.
Department of Physics,
University of Birmingham

ELLIS HORWOOD LIMITED
Publishers · Chichester

Halsted Press: a division of
JOHN WILEY & SONS
New York · Brisbane · Chichester · Toronto

First published in 1981 by
ELLIS HORWOOD LIMITED
Market Cross House, Cooper Street, Chichester, West Sussex, PO19 1EB, England

The publisher's colophon is reproduced from James Gillison's drawing of the ancient Market Cross, Chichester.

Distributors:

Australia, New Zealand, South-east Asia:
Jacaranda-Wiley Ltd., Jacaranda Press,
JOHN WILEY & SONS INC.,
G.P.O. Box 859, Brisbane, Queensland 40001, Australia

Canada:
JOHN WILEY & SONS CANADA LIMITED
22 Worcester Road, Rexdale, Ontario, Canada.

Europe, Africa:
JOHN WILEY & SONS LIMITED
Baffins Lane, Chichester, West Sussex, England.

North and South America and the rest of the world:
Halsted Press: a division of
JOHN WILEY & SONS
605 Third Avenue, New York, N.Y. 10016, U.S.A.

© N. A. Dyson/Ellis Horwood Limited 1981

British Library Cataloguing in Publication Data
Dyson, N. A.
An introduction to nuclear physics, with applications in medicine and biology. –
(Ellis Horwood series in physics in medicine and biology)
1. Nuclear physics
I. Title
539.7'02461   QC776

Library of Congress Card No. 81–6720 AACR2

ISBN 0–85312–265–2 (Ellis Horwood Limited, Publishers – Library Edn.)
ISBN 0–85312–376–4 (Ellis Horwood Limited, Publishers – Student Edn.)
ISBN 0–470–27277–5 (Halsted Press)

Typeset in Press Roman by Ellis Horwood Limited, Publishers
Printed in the U.S.A. by Eastern Graphics Inc., Old Saybrook, Connecticut

AN INTRODUCTION TO NUCLEAR PHYSICS,
WITH APPLICATIONS IN MEDICINE AND BIOLOGY

2

0

Bo

ELLIS HORWOOD SERIES IN MEDICINE AND BIOLOGY

Series Editor:
E. H. GRANT, Professor of Experimental Physics, Queen Elizabeth College, University of London

This series aims to cover ionising radiation and its hazards, the medical and biological effects of radiowaves and microwaves, ultrasonics in medicine and biology, medical imaging, lasers in medicine and biology, and medical electronics. Other books will later be added to the series.

Each book will act as an authoritative guide to its subject and will therefore be appropriate reading for postgraduate students entering its field or for workers in allied fields of research who require information. Practical applications and any attendant hazards will be emphasised and users of apparatus and workers exposed to radiations will therefore find the books a valuable source of knowledge.

Published and in preparation

AN INTRODUCTION TO NUCLEAR PHYSICS,
WITH APPLICATIONS IN MEDICINE AND BIOLOGY
N. A. DYSON, University of Birmingham

IONISING RADIATION AND ITS HAZARDS
R. E. ELLIS, University of Leeds

MICROWAVES AND RADIOWAVES IN MEDICINE AND BIOLOGY
E. H. GRANT, Queen Elizabeth College, University of London

PHYSICAL PRINCIPLES OF MEDICAL ULTRASONICS
C. R. HILL, Institute of Cancer Research, Sutton

Table of Contents

Author's Preface

This book was written to provide a concise account of the applications of nuclear physics to medical and biological science. In order to do this, it seemed necessary to outline some rather basic aspects of nuclear and radiation physics and, in its final form, something approaching half the book is devoted to laying these foundations. The book will therefore be of interest not only to those undergraduates and postgraduates who are devoting their main effort to medical physics, but also to those students who are looking primarily for an introduction to nuclear physics together with an account of some of the ways in which it impinges on the work of other scientists.

The book, then, should appeal to many undergraduates, including those who, in their final year, have selected a biomedical type of option as a means of broadening their scientific interest and also perhaps in order to explore a possible career avenue. The book will also be of value to postgraduates in various disciplines—those who are pursuing post-graduate courses in medical or medically-oriented physics; those who are seeking to become radiobiologists (whether originally students of physics, biology or medicine); and those who, as under-graduates, sought to combine physics with other subjects such as biology or environmental science, and are now needing to develop their nuclear physics to a more useful level than they were able to prior to graduation. Finally, it is hoped that physicists and others who have already embarked on careers in medical physics or environmental science may find the book to be of value.

The *Further Reading* to which the student's attention is particularly drawn, lists those works which for the most part are standard texts in nuclear physics, medical physics, and other more specialised areas of medicine and biology. This book will fulfil one of its purposes if it successfully launches the physicist into a systematic study of the uses of radioisotopes in clinical medicine, or the environmental scientist into the study of the detection and measurement of nuclear radiation. Many of the works listed under this heading contain very extensive lists of references which will assist the reader in his quest for more specialised and detailed material.

I am greatly indebted to Mrs Z. Drolc of the Queen Elizabeth Hospital, Birmingham and to Dr R. G. Harris of the University of Birmingham for reading substantial sections of the text, and for helping me by discussion of the subject matter. Also, I owe a debt to the Series Editor, Professor E. H. Grant, Queen Elizabeth College, University of London, for reading the whole text, and for providing guidance at all stages of preparation. Needless to say, any errors, or infelicities of balance, remain the Author's responsibility. The bulk of the typing was carried out by Mrs Sue Yeomans and Mrs June Layton, to whom my sincere thanks are due.

I am indebted to the following publishers and institutions for permission to reproduce tables and illustrations from their copyright publications: Academic Press Inc., (Fig. 1.2); Cambridge University Press, (Fig. 1.6); Chapman and Hall Ltd., (Fig. 5.5); North Holland Publishing Co., (Figs. 3.9, 3.10, 4.10, 7.2, 7.3); Pergamon Press, (Fig. 4.16); Wiley and Sons, (Fig. 4.4); U.S. Government Printing Office, (Fig. 2.6); also The Institute of Physics (London), The American Institute of Physics. The American Physical Society, and the American Physiological Society. Other acknowledgements appear in the text, and in captions to tables and diagrams. If any acknowledgements have been inadvertently omitted, I shall be glad to be informed, in order to make amends in future printings.

Working on the premise that all ventures of this type can benefit from contact with those for whom the work is intended, the Author would welcome criticisms and suggestions, from readers, whether students, teachers, research workers, or others working in this field, towards improvement of the book in any future edition or reprinting.

N. A. Dyson
University of Birmingham,
April 1981

Glossary of Terms

GLOSSARY OF TERMS

A few terms, both physical and biological, occur in the text at points where an explanation would intrude into the main burden of the argument there, and would cause a digression from the flow of the narrative. Brief explanations of these terms are gathered together here in this short glossary.

Betatron

A cyclic accelerator in which the charged particles are accelerated by a progressively increasing magnetic field perpendicular to the plane of the trajectory. An example of electromagnetic induction operating in the absence of a conductor. Betatrons are used in applied radiation physics for the acceleration of electrons to 20–45 MeV, for Megavoltage radiotherapy.

Bohr Hydrogen Radius

The radius of the electon orbit in the ground state of the hydrogen atom, as evaluated in the treatment due to Bohr. It is given by h^2/me^2 (or, in the form suitable for use with S.I. units, $\epsilon_0 h^2/\pi me^2$) and is equal to 0.529×10^{-10} m.

Bremsstrahlung

When a charged particle is deflected by the Coulomb field of a nucleus, the vector acceleration (or change in direction of velocity vector) can be sufficiently large for radiation of energy to occur, particularly if the moving particle is an electron. This is the mechanism by which the continuous x-ray spectrum is produced by electron bombardment of a target. It occurs to a greater or lesser extent whenever charged particles of any kind interact with matter. A somewhat naive description of the process is to say simply that the process occurs during the slowing-down of the particles, hence the term 'Bremsstrahlung', or 'braking radiation'.

Chemotherapy

The treatment of disease by the administration of chemical agents. In the context of this book it may be contrasted with Radiotherapy, which is the treatment of disease by the use of ionizing radiation.

Cockcroft–Walton generator

A low-energy particle accelerator in which the accelerating field is provided by a voltage-doubler (or quadrupler, etc.) circuit energized by a transformer (usually three-phase) operating at mains frequency.

Coulomb excitation

The raising of a nucleus to an excited state by electromagnetic means, usually by the close passage of a swift charged particle.

Febrile

In medicine, a physiological reaction resulting in a raising of body temperature above normal.

Fermi Energy

In the electron theory of metals, the conduction electrons are shown to occupy a series of levels up to a maximum value which is known as the Fermi Energy. This maximum is sharply-defined at Absolute Zero, becoming somewhat less so as the temperature is raised.

Fluorescence yield

When atoms are ionized in an inner shell, the fluorescence yield is the fraction of such atoms which will emit characteristic x-rays during the subsequent filling of the vacancy, the alternative process being the emission of an Auger electron. The fluorescence yield of the s th shell (where $s = $ K, L, etc.) is thus given by

$$\omega_s = p_x/(p_x + p_a)$$

where p_x and p_a are the probabilities per unit time of x-ray emission and Auger emission respectively.

Half-life: Partial half-life

The half-life is the time taken for a radioactive or otherwise unstable atomic or nuclear species to decay to one-half of its initial activity. The term 'partial half-life' is sometimes used to express the fact that decay may sometimes take place by more than one process, any one of which (if it could occur alone) would give rise to its own characteristic half-life. For example, if the disintegration constant λ of a nuclide decaying by both α-decay and spontaneous fission is given by $\lambda = \lambda_\alpha + \lambda_f$, the quantity $(\ln 2)/\lambda_f$ may be described as the 'fission half-life', or the 'partial half-life with respect to fission'.

Impact Parameter

The perpendicular distance between the line of travel of an initially undeflected particle and the scattering centre (the quantity p in Fig. 1.5 a).

In vitro (Biol.)

An investigation, assay, etc., performed on material of biological origin (which may include living cells) but in inanimate surroundings.

In vivo (Biol.)

An investigation, assay, or other procedure carried out in the living organism or human body.

Isotonic saline

A solution of sodium chloride with the same osmotic pressure as the intracellular fluid. For use in the human body, isotonic saline contains 0.9% NaCl w/w.

Linear Accelerator (or Linac)

A class of particle accelerators in which the charged particles travel in essentially a straight line during the acceleration process (in contrast to *cyclic* accelerators in which the particles describe circular or spiral paths). Although the term was originally applied to relatively low energy accelerators in which the beam passed through a series of drift tubes separated by gaps energised by a radio-frequency field, it is now generally reserved for devices in which the particles ride along a travelling microwave field in what is essentially a waveguide. The length may range from a metre or so, as in the 4 MeV electron linacs used extensively for radiotherapy, to a kilometre or more in accelerators designed to achieve energies of several GeV.

Magic Numbers

In the shell theory of nuclear structure, complete shells occur for certain numbers of nucleons which are given by treatments broadly analogous to the shell theory of electron 'orbits' in atoms. Complete shells confer especial stability of a nucleus, and the *next* nucleon to be added is relatively loosely bound. Complete shells occur when the total numbers of neutrons or protons are equal to 2, 8, 20, 28, 50, 82, and 126. These numbers are known as 'magic' numbers.

Multiplicity

If J is the total angular momentum of an atomic state, the multiplicity is given by $2J + 1$, and similarly for nuclear states of spin I. By the rules of spatial quantization, the multiplicity is the number of orientations available to the total angular momentum vector, and hence it is equal to the number of ways in which a state can be occupied. It follows that it is also the number of levels into which a state can be split by a magnetic field.

Myxoedema

This is a syndrome (group of symptoms) due to **hypothyroidism**, which is underactivity of the thyroid gland resulting in inadequate production of thyroid hormone.

Nucleosynthesis

The process by which the elements may be synthesised from nucleons by successive processes of neutron capture followed by β^--decay. (It may be represented by a 'zig-zag' progress from bottom left to top right in the portion of a Segre chart shown in Fig. 2.3). It is generally conjectured to be the process by which the elements were synthesised from primordial matter. It can also occur for a short period of time in the immediate vicinity of a nuclear explosion, especially when the density of surrounding matter is relatively high (for example, underground).

Parity (with reference to γ-decay processes)

A wave function which retains the same sign under the transformation $x \rightarrow -x$, $y \rightarrow -y$, $z \rightarrow -z$ is said to have **even** parity, and a function which changes sign has **odd** parity. A radiation field possesses the property of parity, and so the process of γ-decay can result in a change of parity of the emitting nucleus, although the parity of the system as a whole (that is, nucleus plus radiation field) is conserved in electromagnetic processes. A γ-transition is therefore specified by a statement of the change, ΔI, of spin, coupled with a statement (Yes or No) of whether the parity of the nucleus changes or not.

pn junction

In semiconductor physics, if an n-type semiconductor (that is, one containing an excess of negative charge carriers) and a p-type (with a deficiency of negative carriers) are placed in contact, a rectifying junction is formed. If it is then biassed in the direction opposite to that which would cause conduction ('reverse-biassed'), any charge carriers in the immediate vicinity of the junction are swept out, and a region of high resistance formed. This is known as a depletion layer. This circumstance is favourable for the detection of ionizing radiation, because the momentary release, in this layer, of electrons, caused by the passage of an ionizing particle will generate an electrical pulse.

Poisson Distribution

In statistics, if there are N_0 opportunities, each with a probability p, for an event to occur, the probability $P(n)$ of n events actually happening is given by the Binomial distribution

$$P(n) = \frac{N_0!}{n!(N_0 - n)!} p^n (1 - p)^{(N_0 - n)}$$

If N_0 is very large and p very small, this expression approaches

$$P(n) = \frac{N^n e^{-N}}{n!}$$

where $N(= N_0 p)$ is the average number of events taking place. This is known as the **Poisson** Distribution, and is relevant to the situation obtaining in radioactive decay, where N_0 is identifiable with the number of radioactive atoms present, and p is the (small) probability of a given atom decaying during an interval of time which is short compared with the half-life. N is therefore the **mean** number of counts occurring during the specified time interval.

Primary biliary cirrhosis

A condition of the liver in which internal changes cause loss of metabolic functions such as the assimilation of copper and other minor elements into essential enzymes. Cirrhosis can be induced as a secondary consequence of external agents such as alcohol or other toxic agents. It is characterised by destruction of normal liver structure and fibrosis.

Right side and left side of the heart

Venous blood, deoxygenated as a result of absorption of oxygen by body tissues enters the right side of the heart, is pumped along the **pulmonary artery** to the lungs, and thence, after becoming oxygenated there, along the **pulmonary veins** to the left side of the heart. From this it emerges into the **aorta** and is transported around the body as oxygenated blood.

Rutherford scattering of charged particles

This is the scattering of positively-charged particles by the electrostatic (Coulomb) field of the nucleus. It was established theoretically, from classical consideration of the movement of particles under central forces, that the differential cross-section for the process should vary as $\mathrm{cosec}^4\,(\theta/2)$, where θ is the scattering angle, and was experimentally verified in many experiments from the time of Rutherford onwards.

Secondary electron emission

When an electron strikes a metallic surface, the kinetic energy is transferred to other electrons, and a few which are close to the surface may be re-emitted. This process is known as secondary emission. The effect becomes appreciable when the energy of the electron exceeds about 50 eV, rises gradually, and then declines for incident energies greater than a few hundred eV. The **secondary emission coefficient** is the ratio of the mean number of secondary electrons emitted per incident electron. A typical maximum value for materials chosen so as to exhibit the effect markedly is in the region of 3. Secondary emission plays an essential role in the operation of the photomultiplier as used in the scintillation counter.

Spallation

The detachment of small parts of a nucleus, or of several individual nucleons, as a result of bombardment by a charged particle of moderately high energy. It is a feature of nuclear reactions at energies above about 40 MeV. (Spall – a splinter or chip, for example, of rock.)

Thermistor

A resistor made with special materials designed to exhibit a large negative temperature coefficient. Used as bridge circuits for the measurement of small temperature changes.

Thyrotoxicosis

This is a syndrome (group of symptoms) due to **hyperthyroidism**, which is overactivity of the thyroid giving rise to excessive production of thyroid hormone.

CHAPTER 1

Interactions between Radiation and Matter

1.1 INTRODUCTORY

In any discussion of the applications of nuclear physics in the fields of medicine and biology, the interaction between ionizing radiation and matter must occupy a place of central importance.

From the earliest days of radiology, some knowledge of the mechanisms by which energy is transmitted through and absorbed by biological tissue was essential, if the image on the photographic emulsion was to be capable of scientific interpretation. Furthermore, the possible therapeutic effects of radiation were soon to be explored, giving rise to the branch of clinical medicine known as radiotherapeutics or, more commonly, radiotherapy. Clearly this depends upon the absorption of radiation by biological tissue, and any calculation of the amount of energy absorbed, or indeed any attempt to measure this quantity experimentally, must involve some knowledge of the physical processes involved. Notice that we have already touched upon two fundamental aspects of radiation interactions – first, the *transmission* of quanta of energy in a well defined radiation beam through a medium to a photographic plate, and secondly, the *absorption* of energy by the irradiated medium. One might be tempted to add, for completeness, that the remaining type of interaction – scattering – has also become of importance in imaging techniques, through the use of the Compton effect, although this development is relatively recent.

These remarks apply to the use of electromagnetic radiation, that is, x-rays and γ-rays. For applications of β-rays in medicine we do not have to seek far – the treatment of skin cancer has for many years been assisted by the availability of β-emitters which can be fabricated into applicators for irradiation purposes. More recently, beams of electrons accelerated to 8 or 10 MeV in linear accelerators have been put into widespread use for radiotherapy, in circumstances where the particular depth–dose distribution offered by such a beam is advantageous. Clearly a full understanding of the potential of these techniques requires a knowledge of the basic interactions between electrons and matter.

Of less obvious interest is the behaviour of alpha-particles in biological tissue. However, in the study of radiological hazards the potential biological effects of α-emitters deposited in the body tissues has to be assessed, and this involves knowing all the physical factors involved in the interaction between the α-particles and the surrounding biological tissue. To cite a further example (to be discussed in Chapter 6), we may note that the biological applications of neutron beams are currently of much interest, and that neutrons transfer energy principally by setting in motion protons, and the nuclei of other light elements. The behaviour of α-particles is clearly relevant here, especially if the experimental and theoretical methods used for the study of α-particles can be applied to the analysis of the behaviour of other light nuclei.

1.2 ENERGY-LOSS OF CHARGED PARTICLES

The energy of a charged particle is lost almost entirely by collision with orbital electrons. To examine this in detail we have to obtain information about the trajectory, as a function of the collision impact parameter, and then we must consider the likely maximum and minimum values of the impact parameter. We need to set up an argument which will cater for a wide range of velocities, and which will be appropriate for both heavy and light particles, for example alpha particles and electrons.

From the simplest considerations it is possible to obtain information of value to us. In a head-on collision between (say) an alpha particle of mass M_α and an electron of mass m, it is easy to show that the maximum energy transferred (Q_0) is $2\,m\mathrm{v}^2$ where v is the velocity of the alpha particle, This may be expressed as

$$Q_0 = 2\,m\mathrm{v}^2 = E_\alpha \frac{4m}{M_\alpha}. \tag{1.1}$$

For a 5 MeV alpha particle this is equal to 2.5 keV. The α-particle therefore loses its energy in small amounts, involving many collisions, before coming to rest. This in turn implies a well-defined range, with little statistical variation from one α-particle to another.

The α-particle may also experience a change of direction as a result of collision with atomic nuclei. This is the well-known *Rutherford scattering*, which is treated in standard texts on nuclear physics (see for example the works listed at the end of this chapter). Although scattering through a large angle is possible, the probability is low, and most scattering events involve a change of direction of much less than one degree. A picture thus emerges of straight tracks, with a well-defined length and little deviation, except perhaps at the very end of the tracks.

When the projectiles consist of electrons the position is different — collision between two particles of equal mass can transfer the whole of the kinetic energy to the stationary particle. Large energy transfers are thus possible, and the path length is much less well-defined. Furthermore, the light particle is much more readily deviated by the nucleus, and so the scattering angles can be large, and the path much more crooked, as a result. It follows that the range of the electron is not necessarily as great as its path-length.

The large transfers of energy which are occasionally possible result in the appearance (in cloud chamber photographs or photographic emulsions) of additional electron tracks branching off the track of the incident particle. These are known as δ-rays, and represent an appreciable fraction ($\approx 30\%$) of the total energy originally present in the incident electron.

We shall see later that an incident electron has the possibility of large angular deflection by nuclear scattering, but with little transfer of energy.

In Appendix 1 we see that an explicit relation between the rate of energy loss (or 'stopping power') and the various parameters may be obtained, which is

$$dE/dx = \left(\frac{1}{4\pi\epsilon_0}\right)^2 \frac{4\pi z^2 e^4 nZ}{mv^2} [\ln \frac{Q_{max}}{\bar{J}} - \ln(1-\beta^2) - \beta^2] \quad (1.2)$$

where the relativistic corrections are appropriate for fast particles. Q_{max} is the maximum energy transferable in a head-on collision, and may range from $2mv^2$ in the case of a heavy incident particle (relativistically, $2m_0v^2/(1-\beta^2)$) to $\frac{1}{2}mv^2$ for an incident electron. m is, in all cases, the electronic rest-mass, and v is the projectile velocity. We note the dependence on z^2, where z is the charge on the projectile. $\bar{J}$ represents, in essence, the *minimum* energy which can be transferred to a bound electron. It is a weighted mean of all the excitation and ionization processes which can occur within the atom and is referred to as the mean excitation/ionization potential for the atom. It is therefore substantially greater than the *least* energy required to ionize an atom, and is not readily relatable to this quantity. It is of the order of 13.5 Z eV. Its presence in a logarithmic term suggests that when the incident particles are electrons (for which Q_{max} is large), the quantity $Q_{max}/\bar{J}$ will be large and therefore that the first logarithmic term will not greatly influence the functional dependence of stopping-power on projectile velocity and target atomic number. For incident α-particles, $Q_{max}/\bar{J}$ is not so large, and the logarithmic term has more effect. In the biophysical field the quantity dE/dx is commonly termed the linear energy transfer (or LET), and we shall have occasion to discuss this aspect later in this book.

1.3 ENERGY-LOSS OF α-PARTICLES

In circumstances where the relativistic corrections may be disregarded, (1.2) reduces to

$$\frac{dE}{dx} = \frac{1}{(4\pi\epsilon_0)^2} \frac{4\pi z^2 e^4}{mv^2} n \left\{ Z \ln \frac{2mv^2}{\bar{J}} \right\}. \quad (1.3)$$

n may be written as $N_A \rho \dfrac{Z}{A}$, where N_A is Avogadro's number and ρ the density of the material, so we may write

$$\frac{dE}{d(\rho x)} = \frac{1}{(4\pi\epsilon_0)^2} \frac{4\pi z^2 e^4}{m v^2} N_A \frac{Z}{A} \ln \frac{2m v^2}{\bar{J}}$$

$$= \frac{1}{(4\pi\epsilon_0)^2} \frac{2\pi z^2 e^4}{E_\alpha} \frac{M_\alpha}{m} N_A \frac{Z}{A} \ln \frac{4E_\alpha}{\bar{J}} \frac{m}{M_\alpha}. \qquad (1.4)$$

$dE/d(\rho x)$ is termed the *specific energy loss*, and may be denoted by S. The charge z on the projectile is now 2 units of electronic charge.

This expression is useful for α-particles with energies greater than about 2 MeV. Below this energy the effective z of the projectile becomes progressively less than 2 because of increasing charge exchange between the slowly-moving α-particle and the electronic cloud through which it moves.

Furthermore, the binding energies of some of the orbital electrons may exceed $E_\alpha \dfrac{4m}{M_\alpha}$ (see equation 1.1) leading to inability of these electrons to participate in the slowing down process. This non-participation may be allowed for by subtracting a term $C_{K,L}$ from the part of the expression in (1.2), which we have enclosed in square brackets. This treatment is described by Evans (1955).

Both these factors give rise to a reduced value of specific energy loss at low particle energies.

The variation of specific energy loss with energy is illustrated in Fig. 1.1. The

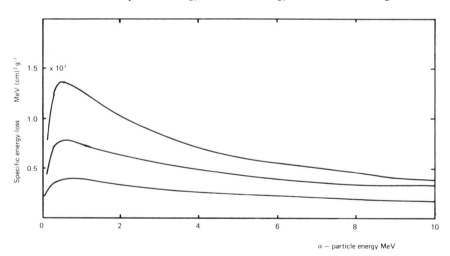

Fig. 1.1 Specific energy-loss of α-particles as a function of energy.
(From the data of Williamson *et al.* (1976))

approximately $1/E_\alpha$ dependence expected from equation (1.4) is partially offset by the effect of the logarithmic term. Empirically, the specific energy loss of α-particles of energy in the region of a few MeV (as encountered in radioactive decay) has been found to vary approximately as $E^{-\frac{1}{2}}$. This enables us to perform an integration to obtain the range as a function of energy

$$\frac{\mathrm{d}E}{\mathrm{d}(\rho x)} = kE^{-\frac{1}{2}}. \tag{1.5}$$

Hence $(\rho x)_0 = \dfrac{2k^{-1}}{3} E_\alpha^{\frac{3}{2}}$, where $(\rho x)_0$ is the distance travelled by the α-particle in order to bring it to rest. It may be denoted by R. This is known as *Geiger's rule*, and is applicable to α-particles of 4-10 MeV.

Similarly the variation with Z or A is not expressible in simple form. Equation (1.4) indicates that the specific energy loss will fall slightly with increasing Z, because the quantity Z/A diminishes slowly, and $\bar{J}$ increases steadily, as Z is increased. The "mass–range", R, of α-particles (i.e. the range expressed in terms of mass per unit area) is thus expected to increase with atomic weight or atomic number, and the empirical expression

$$R_1 : R_2 = \sqrt{A_1} : \sqrt{A_2} \tag{1.6}$$

has been found useful. This is known as the Bragg-Kleeman rule.

Much tabulated data on stopping powers and ranges is available in the literature. Some data for "mass-range" as a function of E and Z, for α-particles, are shown in Table 1.1. The range of a 5 MeV α-particle in biological tissue is in the region of 40 μm.

Table 1.1

Range of α-particles as a function of atomic number and α-particle energy
(from the data of Williamson *et al.*, 1966)

Energy in MeV	Carbon	Oxygen	Aluminium	Copper	Silver	Gold	Uranium
			Range in mg (cm)$^{-2}$				
0.2	0.262	0.319	0.449	0.726	0.932	1.19	1.28
0.5	0.376	0.456	0.648	1.09	1.43	1.91	2.07
1.0	0.588	0.705	0.994	1.69	2.28	3.12	3.43
1.5	0.849	1.003	1.39	2.36	3.21	4.47	4.95
2	1.16	1.35	1.85	3.11	4.25	5.97	6.62
3	1.94	2.21	2.94	4.82	6.59	9.34	10.4
4	2.91	3.28	4.25	6.81	9.27	13.2	14.7
6	5.40	5.98	7.53	11.6	15.5	22.1	24.7
8	8.59	9.41	11.6	17.3	22.9	32.4	36.3

Because the nature of the processes by which α-particles lose energy is essentially statistical, the range is not completely uniform, but is subject to a small statistical variation known as 'straggling' or 'range-straggling'. This variation is in the region of 1%. It is observed in the case of all heavy particles, including fission fragments, although in the latter case the possibility of nuclear reactions increases the straggling.

A curve of great relevance in the present context is the ionization curve or 'Bragg' curve. This is closely related to the varying value of dE/dx as the particle is slowed down and reveals, as we would expect, a peak in ionization density towards the end of the range. The effect of the progressive change in dE/dx is modified somewhat by the straggling, increasing the width of the ionization peak and providing a 'tail' at the end of the range. The peak of ionization at the end of the track is illustrated in Fig. 1.2.

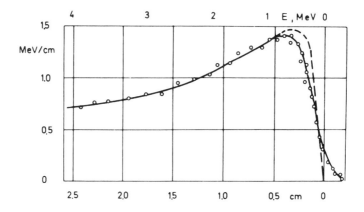

Fig. 1.2   The 'Bragg curve' (experimental points) for α-particles, showing ionization per unit length as a function of distance travelled in air. (The dotted curve shows the ionization curve of a single particle.) (Mladjenović, 1973)

The scattering of α-particles usually involves very small angles, and, although large-angle scattering is of the greatest significance in evaluating the Rutherford scattering theory, the contribution to the loss of α-particles from a parallel beam is small. We may plot a "number–distance" curve shown schematically in Fig. 1.3, in which the curve is flat until the end of the range is approached, when range-straggling (and the occasional large angle scattering event — somewhat more likely when the kinetic energy has been reduced to a low value) begins to reduce the number of particles in the beam.

We shall see that this behaviour contrasts very sharply with the behaviour of electrons, which we discuss in the next three sections.

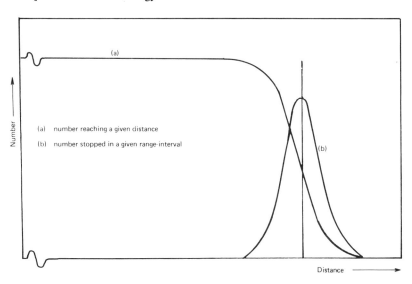

Fig. 1.3 'Number–distance' curve for α-particles

1.4 ENERGY-LOSS FROM ELECTRON BEAMS

Electrons encountered in radioactive decay are normally swifter than the α-particles discussed in the foregoing section, and so we must be prepared for a wider range of velocities, extending well into the relativistic region. Equation (1.2) will continue to serve us, bearing in mind that $z = 1$ and that Q_{max} is now equal to the full energy of the incident electron. There are, however, small differences in the logarithmic term, partly because the projectile and 'target' are now identical particles, and also because the reduced mass of the two electrons must be brought into the calculation. For example, for non-relativistic electrons,

$$\frac{dE}{dx} = \frac{1}{(4\pi\epsilon_0)^2} \frac{4\pi e^4 n Z}{mv^2} \ln \frac{kmv^2}{2\bar{J}} \tag{1.7}$$

where k is variously given as $\sqrt{2}$ (Evans, 1955) or $(e/2)^{1/2}$ (Segrè, 1977).

Because of the much greater velocity of β-particles, the logrithmic term in (1.7) is greater, and its variation with E and Z therefore less, than in equation (1.3) for α-particles.

For certain purposes it is convenient to write (1.7) in the form

$$\frac{dE}{dx} = \frac{1}{(4\pi\epsilon_0)^2} \frac{4\pi e^4}{mv^2} nB, \tag{1.8}$$

where B is the *stopping number*. This indicates that for non-relativistic electrons the stopping power is expected to vary as $1/E$. If the reciprocal of this is integrated to obtain the integrated path length R, for electrons of initial energy E_0 and initial velocity V_0, neglecting variation of B with energy, we obtain

$$R = \int_{E_0}^{0} \left| \frac{dx}{dE} \right| dE = \text{const} \times E_0^2 \qquad (1.9)$$

This proportionality with E_0^2 (or v_0^4) has been known for a long time in the case of low energy electrons (for example electrons in discharge tubes or x-ray tubes) and is known as the Thomson–Whiddington law. It is approximately true for electrons less than about 50 keV in energy. At higher energies. the velocity begins to rise less rapidly on account of relativity, so the 'square–law' relationship falls off.

At still higher energies the stopping power becomes approximately independent of energy, and the range in consequence varies approximately linearly with energy. A graph of range *versus* energy is shown in Fig. 1.4. This represents the combined data of many workers, for details of which the original reference may be consulted. The data were obtained using light elements as absorbers, and illustrate that the range is approximately independent of atomic number for

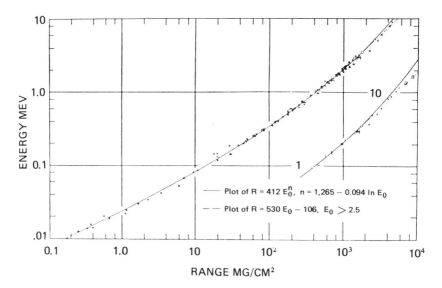

Fig. 1.4 Range/energy relation for electrons in light elements ($Z \leqslant 13$). Some empirical expressions for range, devised to fit the experimental points, are also given (after Katz and Penfold, 1952)

$Z \lesssim 13$, However, an electron suffers some scattering during the slowing-down process, and so it follows that the range will be less than the integrated path length by a significant amount. For example, in aluminium the ratio of the former to the latter varies between about 0.45 and 0.7 for electron energies in the energy-range 10–70 keV.

At higher atomic numbers, the path becomes more crooked and these ratios are therefore even less. Therefore, although the integrated path length increases appreciably with atomic number, the range varies only slightly.

The approximately linear variation of range with energy for electrons of energy greater than about 3 MeV is consistent with data on the radiation dose (*q.v.*) delivered to water or biological tissue by collimated beams of electrons, obtained from linear accelerators and betatrons designed for use in the field of radiotherapy.

Empirical relationships such as

$$R = \frac{E}{2} - \frac{1}{2} \ (R \text{ in cm. of water}, E \text{ in MeV}) \tag{1.10}$$

tending to $\ R = E/2$ (1.11)

at higher energies are found to be of practical use.

1.5 RADIATIVE LOSSES FOR ELECTRONS

In addition to the energy-loss described in the previous section, radiative losses also occur. These are the processes which are responsible for the production of the continuous x-ray spectrum, or Bremsstrahlung, in x-ray tubes. Their origin can be found in classical electrodynamics. where it is shown that any accelerated charge will radiate energy at a rate depending upon the magnitudes of the charge and the acceleration. An electron interacting with the coulomb field of a nucleus will experience an acceleration sufficiently large to cause radiation, although the classical concept of radiation *at a mean rate* must be replaced by a quantum–mechanical *probability* of a photon being emitted; an electron may not radiate at all, or may radiate a substantial amount of energy in a single interaction.

The acceleration produced at a distance r from the nucleus will be equal to the force divided by the electronic mass, i.e.

$$a = \frac{1}{4\pi\epsilon_0} \frac{Ze^2}{mr^2}, \tag{1.12}$$

and the rate at which energy is radiated will be proportional the square of this quantity. This leads to a radiative cross-section proportional to Z^2. This may be compared with the ionization cross-section per atom, which is proportional to the number of electrons per atom, i.e., to Z. We therefore expect radiative losses to be relatively more important at higher atomic numbers.

For the energy-loss by radiation

$$
\left.
\begin{aligned}
E_{\text{rad}}\,dx\,dv &= \frac{Z^2 n\,dx\,dv}{E} \quad (v < v_0) \\[2ex]
&= 0 \quad\quad\quad (v > v_0)
\end{aligned}
\right\}
\tag{1.13}
$$

This is essentially a 'white–noise' spectrum with a quantum cut-off at $v = v_0$, the high frequency limit, given by $hv_0 = E$, the energy of the electron. Integrating from v_0 to 0,

$$
dE_{\text{rad}} = E_{\text{rad}}\,dx = \frac{Z^2 n v_0\,dx}{E} = \frac{Z^2 n\,dx}{h}
\tag{1.14}
$$

i.e. dE_{rad} is the radiative energy-loss per electron in a thickness dx, for an electron of energy E.

For ionization losses we write

$$
\frac{dE_{\text{ion}}}{dx} = \frac{\text{const.} \times Zn}{E}
\tag{1.15}
$$

or $\quad\quad dE_{\text{ion}} = \text{const.} \times \dfrac{Zn}{E}.dx$

Hence we can write

$$
\left(\frac{dE}{dx}\right)_{\text{rad}} \bigg/ \left(\frac{dE}{dx}\right)_{\text{ion}} \propto ZE
\tag{1.16}
$$

At relativistic energies, the energy losses given by (1.13) and (1.15) both become more nearly independent of E, but the ratio given in (1.16) remains approximately proportional to E, and to Z.

For lead ($Z = 82$) the two mechanisms for energy-loss become equal at about 9 MeV. For water or air, the corresponding energy lies in the region of 100 MeV. For electrons of less than 1 MeV the radiative energy loss will not exceed a few percent of the energy losses by other processes. This begins to be important to us, however, in radiation dosimetry, where it becomes apparent that when evaluating the absorbed dose from fast electrons, a correction has to be applied to allow for loss of energy from the system by Bremsstrahlung.

1.6 ELECTRON SCATTERING

The mechanisms by which electrons lose energy by interaction with matter have been discussed, but a further interaction requires consideration — the interaction with atomic nuclei. Simple kinetic considerations show that the change of energy in such an encounter is very small indeed, and can be neglected when evaluating energy-loss from an electron. However, the scattering is significant, both in the magnitude of the scattering angle and in the probability for the process to occur.

If we consider the problem in the manner depicted in Fig. 1.5, we can apply the analysis used for the Rutherford scattering of α-particles, and can write

$$p = \frac{b}{2} \cot \frac{\theta}{2} \tag{1.17}$$

where
$$b = \frac{2Ze^2}{m\mathrm{v}^2} \tag{1.18}$$

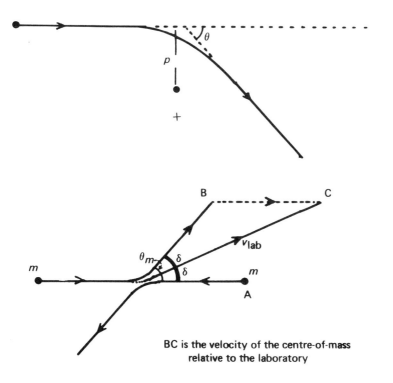

BC is the velocity of the centre-of-mass relative to the laboratory

Fig. 1.5 (a) Classical trajectory of an electron in the coulomb field of a nucleus. (b) Classical trajectories illustrating electron–electron scattering, in laboratory and in centre-of-mass coordinates

Because the ratio of nuclear to electron masses is very large, the centre-of-mass system resembles closely the laboratory system, and no transformation into the latter is necessary.

Equations (1.17) and (1.18) lead directly to

$$\tan \frac{\theta}{2} = \frac{Ze^2}{2E\rho}$$

$$\text{or} \quad \theta \sim \frac{Ze^2}{E\rho} \qquad (1.19)$$

For an electron/electron encounter, we may write

$$b = \frac{2e^2}{M_0 v^2}$$

where M_0 is the reduced mass of the electron/electron system ($= m/2$), and from (1.17),

$$\tan \frac{\theta_m}{2} = \frac{b}{2p},$$

remembering that θ_m is in the centre-of-mass system.

Hence $\qquad \tan \dfrac{\theta_m}{2} = \dfrac{e^2}{E\rho},$

and, from Fig. 1.15 (b)

$$\delta = \frac{\theta_m}{2}$$

Hence $\qquad \delta = \dfrac{\theta_m}{2} = \dfrac{e^2}{E\rho}, \qquad (1.20)$

which is less than θ in (1.19) by a factor of Z. Therefore the nuclear scattering angles may be expected to be $\sim Z$ times greater than those resulting from electron/electron collisions.

The collision energy-loss in nuclear collisions is given by

$$\Delta E = 4E \frac{m}{M} \sin^2 \frac{\theta}{2}, \qquad (1.21)$$

whereas in electron/electron collisions

$$\Delta E = E \sin^2 \delta \tag{1.22}$$

Hence $$\frac{\Delta E_{\text{el-el}}}{\Delta E_{\text{el-nucl}}} = \frac{\sin^2 \delta}{4 \frac{m}{M} \sin^2 \frac{\theta}{2}} \approx \frac{M}{m} \left(\frac{\delta}{\theta} \right)^2, \tag{1.23}$$

for small angles.

For equal impact parameters, this may be written as

$$\frac{M}{m} \frac{1}{Z^2} \tag{1.24}$$

Bearing in mind that there are Z electrons per atom, we have

$$\frac{\Delta E_{\text{el-el}}}{\Delta E_{\text{el-nucl}}} \approx \frac{M}{m} \frac{1}{Z}, \text{ which is} \gg 1. \tag{1.25}$$

We may therefore conclude that encounters with nuclei are primarily responsible for *scattering*, and encounters with electrons cause *energy-loss*. This important generalization is the key to elucidating many features of the behaviour of electron beams in matter.

The cross-section for elastic (nuclear) scattering may be expected to vary as Z^2 (Rutherford scattering law) whereas the inelastic (electron) cross-section per atom will vary simply as Z. The elastic process will become relatively more important at high Z, and detailed considerations show that it is also in fact numerically greater. The two processes are equally probable at $Z \approx 30$ (Lenz, 1954), and in light elements the inelastic process has the greater probability.

We can now assert that the ratio of range to integrated path length may be expected to fall steadily as Z is increased, and this is found to be the case in practice. Furthermore, if we consider the problem of experimentally measuring the counting rate when an electron beam travels through varying thicknesses of matter to a detector (for example a Geiger counter) we may expect differences in the transmission curves. In the case of a light element, scattering angles tend to be small, and scattering events infrequent; several scattering events will be needed to remove an electron from the beam, if reasonably broad-beam geometry prevails. The curve will fall off very slowly at first and then more rapidly as the absorber thickness is increased. Curves such as the one for Al in Fig. 1.6, and the curves in Fig. 1.7, are the result. On the other hand, if the absorber is a high-Z material, a single collision will be sufficient to remove an electron from the beam, and we would expect a function which is exponential in form to result from this. The high-Z curve in Fig. 1.6 illustrates this point. It is clear that range as such becomes progressively more difficult to define as Z is increased, and that the

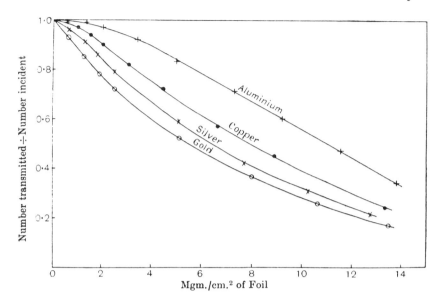

Fig. 1.6 The transmission of electrons (146 keV) through foils of several elements
(Eddy, 1929)

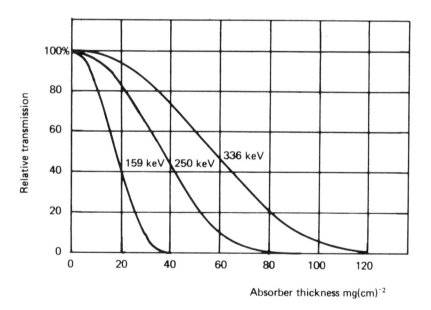

Fig. 1.7 The transmission of electrons through aluminium at 3 different energies
(Seliger, 1955)

behaviour of the beam might better be described in terms of a mean free path, or linear absorption coefficient. This approach is found to be of value in some circumstances.

1.7 INTERACTION BETWEEN γ-RADIATION
AND MATTER-INTRODUCTION

We have seen how a charged particle loses energy by many collisions, each resulting in only a small energy-loss. With gamma-rays the situation is different. An interaction between a photon of γ-radiation and matter can result in a substantial transfer of energy, or even complete absorption of the photon. Alternatively, the photon may be scattered rather than absorbed, that is may experience a change in direction whilst remaining unchanged in energy.

We must note carefully the distinction between the processes which actually transfer energy from radiation to matter, and those which merely change the direction of photons incident on the atom with which they are interacting. That is, we must distinguish between *absorption* and *scattering*, and we must also be able to describe situations in which there is partial absorption of the energy of an incident photon, the remainder appearing as electromagnetic radiation of lower photon energy. We note, however, that all these processes will remove a photon from a beam of photons incident upon matter, and so the *attenuation* of a beam will be a feature of all interactions.

To describe the probability of an interaction occurring, we define a *cross-section* for the process. This is an 'effective area' presented by an atom to the incident beam, and if the matter consists of a foil of a atoms (of one kind) per unit volume, with thickness dx, we see that the number of atoms per unit area presented to the beam is $a\,dx$, and, if the 'removal cross-section' is denoted by σ we can write

$$\frac{dN}{N} = -\sigma a\,dx$$

where N is the number of photons in the primary beam.

Integrating the thickness from 0 to x, we get

$$N = N_0 e^{-a\sigma x} \qquad (1.26)$$

representing the exponential removal of photons from the parallel beam incident upon the foil. This exponential feature is characteristic of the attenuation of a beam of γ-radiation, and is not observed in the case of charged particles, except in the rather special circumstances referred to at the end of section 1.6.

The quantity $a\sigma$ in (1.26) is often written as Σ, the macroscopic cross-section, or as μ, the linear attenuation coefficient. The former terminology has developed mainly in the field of neutron physics, and the latter in the physics of x-rays and γ-rays. The quantity σ is commonly measured in units of 1 barn ($10^{-28}\,m^2$). It may be very small (millibarns) compared with atomic dimensions, if the removal process occurs with only a very small probability; or it may be comparable with atomic dimensions ($\sim 10^{-20}\,m^2$) if the probability is large. It would not surprise us if the square of the *wavelength of the incident radiation* turned out to be as important as the physical dimension of the atoms involved in the interaction process.

1.8 THE PHOTOELECTRIC PROCESS

This consists of the ejection of a bound electron from an inner shell of an atom. If the binding energy is E_x (for the xth shell; $x = K, L, M$, etc.) and the photon energy E_γ, we can write, for the kinetic energy of the ejected electron

$$E_\gamma - E_x$$

The overriding requirement for the interaction that $E_\gamma > E_x$. This gives rise to the absorption edges which are apparent in Fig. 1.8. The proabability of

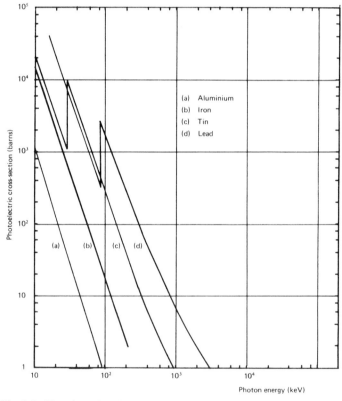

Fig. 1.8 The photoelectric cross-section for several elements, as a function of the photon energy

the process occurring may be understood qualitatively by means of the concept of 'oscillator strength', as developed by, for example, James (1967). The observed dependence on E_γ and Z is not simple, but is found to be of the form

$$\tau \propto Z^\alpha E^{-\beta} \tag{1.27}$$

where α lies between 4 and 5, and β is approximately 3. We thus observe a strong dependence on atomic number (corresponding to an increase in the oscillator strength for a given frequency as Z is increased) and a strong inverse dependence on photon energy (because the oscillator strength falls rapidly as the oscillator frequency is increased).

Photoelectric absorption therefore has some of the qualities of a resonant process, and the absorption edge may be schematically depicted as consisting of a continuum of resonant peaks (Fig. 1.9). This aspect of the photoelectric

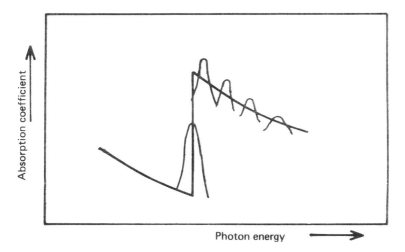

Fig. 1.9 Schematic representation of photoelectric absorption as the sum of a continuum of resonant peaks

process is of no concern when considering photoelectric absorption, but is relevant when the influence of the photoelectric process upon γ-ray scattering is being considered. The oscillators are capable of scattering radiation, and this scattered radiation is coherent with the radiation scattered by Rayleigh scattering (see section 1.10). The phase of the resonantly-scattered radiation changes from 0 to $-\pi$ radians as the resonance is traversed, introducing an anomaly into the amplitude of the scattered radiation in the vicinity of the adsorption edge of the scattering element. This *anomalous* scattering is observed in x-ray diffractometry, and gives strong support to the treatment of the photoelectric absorption in terms of oscillator strengths.

When the incident γ-radiation has a photon energy just below the K absorption discontinuity, the main absorption mechanism is provided by the L electrons. Because the electron density of the L electrons close to the nucleus (that is near the K orbit) is mainly provided by the 2s electrons, and because the value of the square of the wave-amplitude* of those electrons is only about 1/8 of that of the K electrons, the magnitude of the absorption discontinuity is expected to be of the order of 8:1. This is observed to be true in practice for elements in the middle range of Z. A few values of the 'K-jump' are tabulated in Table 1.2.

Table 1.2

Values of mass attenuation coefficients at the K absorption edge,
for a few elements

Z	Edge (KeV)	Total (cm² g⁻¹)			Photoelectric only (cm² g⁻¹)		
		upper	lower	ratio	upper	lower	ratio
13 Al	1.559	4300	370	11.6			
22 Ti	4.96	690	83	8.3			
26 Fe	7.11	(470)	53	8.8			
29 Cu	8.98	306	38	8.1			
42 Mo	20.00	83.9	12.8	6.6	82.8	11.7	7.1
50 Sn	29.19	46.4	7.87	5.9	45.7	7.11	6.4
74 W	69.51	11.4	2.55	4.5	11.0	2.15	5.1
82 Pb	88.00	8.01	1.85	4.4	7.68	1.52	5.1

The strong Z-dependence of photoelectric adsorption is an essential basis of diagnostic radiology, in which the transmission of x-rays through the body enables internal structures to be imaged on a fluorescent screen or photographic film. The degree of absorption at any point in the body is determined by the density and the atomic number of the material at that point. Furthermore, the continuous x-ray spectrum favoured generally for radiography contains a wide range of photon energies, so that the strong energy-dependence of the photoelectric absorption ensures that the absorption cross-sections also extend over a wide range. This allows detail to be imaged effectively in both lightly-absorbing and strongly-absorbing anatomical features. X-ray tubes for diagnostic work are

$$* \quad \psi^2(0) \text{ for an s electron } = \left. \begin{array}{l} \dfrac{4}{\pi} G^2 e^{-2x} \quad \text{(K shell)} \\[2ex] \dfrac{4}{\pi} G^2 e^{-2x} (1-x)^2 \quad \text{(L shell)} \\[2ex] \dfrac{4}{3\pi} G^2 e^{-2x} \left(1 - 2x + \dfrac{2}{3} x^2\right)^2 \quad \text{(M shell)} \end{array} \right\} \quad (1.28)$$

where $G^2 = (Z/na_H)^3$, $x = rZ/na_H$ and $n = 1, 2, 3$ for the K, L and M shells. These expressions need to be doubled to allow for the fact that there are two of these electrons present in each case.

normally limited to potentials of 90–100 kV, imposing a corresponding limit on the photon energies present in the spectrum. If higher photon energies were used, other interaction processes, in particular the Compton effect (to be described in section 1.9), would become important. The Compton effect has a much reduced Z-dependence, and also gives rise to considerable scattered radiation. Both of these effects would cause the contrast in the image, and hence the visibility of many of its features, to be greatly reduced.

1.9 THE COMPTON EFFECT

So far we have considered the behaviour of relatively stongly-bound electrons in the field of an incident beam of γ-radiation. We must now consider the behaviour of free, or weakly bound, electrons. Such electrons are able to interact with a photon of γ-radiation in accordance with the laws of conservation of momentum and energy. Referring to Fig. 1.10 we may write down equations as follows:

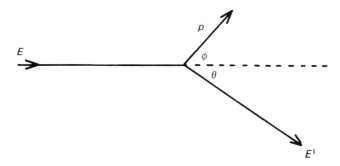

Fig. 1.10 Illustrating the Compton effect

For the conservation of momentum:

$$p \sin \phi = \frac{E'}{c} \sin \theta \tag{1.29a}$$

$$E/c = p \cos \phi + \frac{E'}{c} \cos \theta \tag{1.29b}$$

For the conservation of energy:

$$U^2 = p^2 c^2 + m_0^2 c^4$$

Hence $$T(T + 2m_0 c^2) = p^2 c^2 \tag{1.30a}$$

and also $$E - E' = T \tag{1.30b}$$

From (1.29) and (1.30)

$$p^2 = \left(\frac{E'}{c}\right)^2 \sin \theta + \frac{1}{c^2} (E - E' \cos \theta)^2 \qquad (1.31)$$

and

$$p^2 = \frac{1}{c^2} (E - E')(E - E' + 2m_0c^2) \qquad (1.32)$$

Eliminating p between (1.31) and (1.32), it is readily shown that

$$\frac{1}{E'} - \frac{1}{E} = \frac{1}{m_0c^2} (1 - \cos \theta). \qquad (1.33)$$

A photon is therefore scattered by the electron with a change of energy, and this is a function of the scattering angle. This may be calculated from (1.33), but may be seen more clearly as a change (increase) of wavelength given by

$$\lambda' - \lambda = \frac{h}{m_0c} (1 - \cos \theta) \qquad (1.34)$$

In this equation, h/m_0c is known as the *Compton wavelength*, and is equal to 2.426×10^{-12} m. Radiation with wavelength much greater than this (corresponding to $E_\gamma \ll 511$ KeV) suffers a relatively small fractional change in photon energy (or wavelength). Radiation with a wavelength much *shorter* (that is $E_\gamma \gg 511$ KeV) has an increment added to it which causes the scattered radiation to approach a constant wavelength (irrespective of the value of the primary wavelength) which, for 90° scattering, approaches 2.426×10^{-12}m or 511 keV. For 180° scattering, the wavelength approaches a value of twice, and the photon energy one-half, of this amount.

Much of the γ-radiation encountered in applied radiation physics and medical physics does not conveniently approach these limiting categories, and we may display the *scattered* versus *incident* photon energy, as shown in Fig. 1.11. The limiting case of 180° scattering is important for problems of radiation detection and radiation shielding and we see that, for a wide range of photon energies encountered in practice (500 keV–5 MeV) this scattered radiation lies in the vicinity of 200 keV. Compton scattering tends to be in this region of photon energy, and the radiation is then further degraded (though in smaller steps) by further Compton scattering processes until it can be absorbed by the photoelectric process.

We have not yet discussed the Compton process in terms of a cross-section. As the Compton effect is concerned with free electrons, we might expect the cross section for Compton scattering to be of the order of the square of the classical electron radius, r_e. *

$r_e = \dfrac{1}{4\pi\epsilon_0} \dfrac{e^2}{mc^2}$ or $\dfrac{\mu_0}{4\pi} \dfrac{e^2}{m}$. This quantity is equal to 2.818×10^{-15} m.

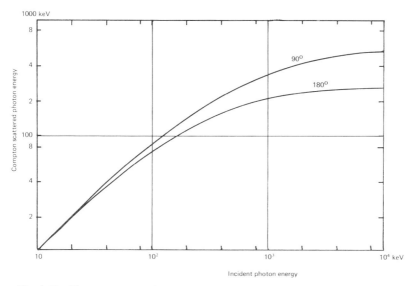

Fig. 1.11　Photon energy after Compton scattering as a function of incident photon energy

The cross-section for Compton interaction with a free electron has been analysed by Klein and Nishina, and detailed accounts of this work, together with graphs and formula, have been given by, for example Evans (1955). It is not part of the present scheme to give a detailed description of this, but for reference purposes a few of the somewhat complicated expressions are given in Appendix 2. At low frequencies, the cross-section per electron (integrated over all scattering angles and assuming unpolarised radiation) is given approximately by

$$\sigma = \frac{8}{3}\pi r_e^2 (1 - 2\alpha) \tag{1.35}$$

where r_e is the classical electron radius, and α is equal to E_γ/mc^2. The Klein–Nishina cross-section per electron is illustrated, as a function of photon energy, in Fig. 1.12. However, a more detailed consideration of the problem has shown that below a certain photon energy an atomic electron may no longer be regarded as free. Its contribution to Compton scattering therefore diminishes, and this is also illustrated in Fig. 1.12.

Compton scattering is an 'incoherent' scattering process, in which all atomic electrons act independently. The *atomic* cross-section for Compton scattering is thus equal to Z times the Klein–Nishina cross section, diminished at low photon energies by the effect of atomic binding.

In the next section we shall see that a bound electron is able to scatter electromagnetic radiation by a process which is most easily discussed classically.

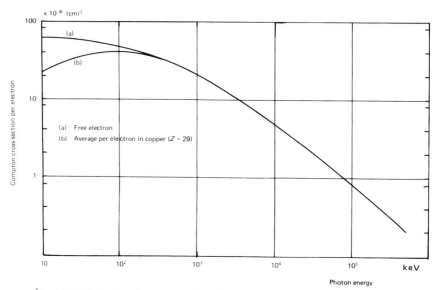

Fig. 1.12 Illustrating the cross-section for Compton scattering with correction for binding energy

1.10 THOMSON AND RAYLEIGH SCATTERING

In this section we consider the behaviour of an electron interacting with γ-radiation at low photon energies (low frequencies). We consider the electron to be capable of vibrating (that is executing forced harmonic motion) under the influence of the field of the incident electromagnetic wave. We note that this approach neglects all consideration of the momentum of the incident radiation. But we may also note that if the electron is bound to an atom, the incident momentum will be transferred to the atom as a whole, with the absorption of very little energy, remembering that $E = p^2/2M$, where M is now an *atomic* rather than *electronic* mass. Virtually the whole of the energy of the incident photon remains available for the scattered photon, and an elastic scattering process becomes possible.

Consider the free electron in Fig. 1.13, irradiated by electromagnetic radiation, which is plane-polarised with its electric vector in the plane of the diagram. Let the incident electric field strength be E_i, and the scattered field strength at a distance r from the electron be E_s. We shall be concerned with the energy flux per unit time associated with these fields, which is given by the Poynting vector for an electromagnetic wave, $W = E \times H$, which, if E and H are at right-angles and in phase, leads directly to an energy flux, averaged over a large number of periods of the electromagnetic wave, given by

$$\langle W \rangle = \langle E^2 \rangle \epsilon_0 c \qquad (1.36)$$

where ϵ_0 is the permittivity of free space and c the velocity of light.

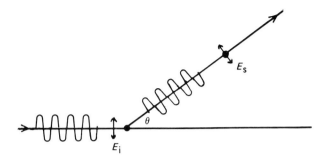

Fig. 1.13 Thomson scattering

The energy scattered in a time dt across an area dS, distance r from the electron, may be written as

$$\langle E_s^2 \rangle \, \epsilon_0 c \, dS \, dt, \tag{1.37a}$$

or $\qquad \langle E_s^2 \rangle \, \epsilon_0 c r^2 \, d\omega \, dt.$ (1.37b)

If we suppose that the scatterer contains just one electron per unit area, the energy represented by (1.37) may also be written as the incident energy flux multiplied by the *differential* cross-section of the electron effective in scattering into the solid angle $d\omega$, that is, as

$$\langle E_i^2 \rangle \, \epsilon_0 c \, d\sigma \, dt \tag{1.38}$$

The differential cross-section for scattering into a solid angle $d\omega$ is thus given by

$$d\sigma = \frac{\langle E_s^2 \rangle}{\langle E_i^2 \rangle} r^2 \, d\omega \tag{1.39}$$

To obtain $\langle E_s^2 \rangle$ we need to use a result from classical electrodynamics which states that the field strength E_s at a distance r from an accelerated charge e is given by

$$E_s = \frac{1}{4\pi\epsilon_0} \frac{ea}{rc^2} \cos\theta \tag{1.40}$$

where a is the acceleration of the electron and θ the angle shown in Fig. 1.13. In the present circumstances

$$a = \frac{E_i e}{m}$$

Hence $\qquad E_s = \dfrac{1}{4\pi\epsilon_0} \dfrac{e^2}{mrc^2} . E_i \cos\theta,$ $\qquad\qquad\qquad$ (1.41)

and the differential cross-section thus becomes (from (1.39) and (1.41)),

$$d\sigma = \frac{1}{(4\pi\epsilon_0)^2} \left(\frac{e^2}{mc^2}\right)^2 \cos^2\theta . d\omega$$

$$= r_e^2 \cos^2\theta \, d\omega \qquad\qquad\qquad (1.42)$$

where r_e is once again the classical electron radius. If the polarisation of the incident radiation is perpendicular to the plane of Fig. 1.13 all the rays scattered in the plane of the diagram are perpendicular to the acceleration of the electron so we may replace $\cos\theta$ by 1. For unpolarised radiation, which is the most common situation in applied radiation physics, we must take the average value, which is $\frac{1}{2}(1 + \cos^2\theta)$.

Hence $\qquad d\sigma = \frac{1}{2}r_e^2(1 + \cos^2\theta) \, d\omega,$ $\qquad\qquad\qquad$ (1.43)

and, if we integrate over all values of θ to obtain the total cross section, we obtain

$$\sigma = r_e^2 \int_{-\frac{\pi}{2}}^{+\frac{\pi}{2}} 2\pi \sin\theta \, (1 + \cos^2\theta) \, d\theta = \frac{8}{3}\pi r_e^2. \qquad (1.44)$$

This is the value to which the Klein–Nishina cross-section tends at low photon energies, showing that the two treatments are mutually consistent in the classical limit. Its value is 0.66×10^{-28} m^2, or 0.66 barn.

It must be stressed that the atomic binding effects referred to in the previous section reduce the Compton cross-section below its Klein–Nishina value, and that this effect becomes more marked as the atomic number increases. The change in the relative importance of the two processes is illustrated in Fig. 1.14, in the case of scattering of silver characteristic radiation from a series of elements.

When considering scattering from atoms (as distinct from free electrons), it is necessary to note that the Thomson scattering from all the individual electrons in the atom is coherent. This implies that the amplitudes of the scattered waves have to be added before squaring to give the intensity (or cross-section). The scattering cross-section in the forward direction is therefore proportional to Z^2. This is in clear contrast to the Z dependence of the Compton process.

The second consequence to stem from the coherence of the elastically-scattered component is that in all directions other than the forward direction the scattered waves interfere destructively to some extent.

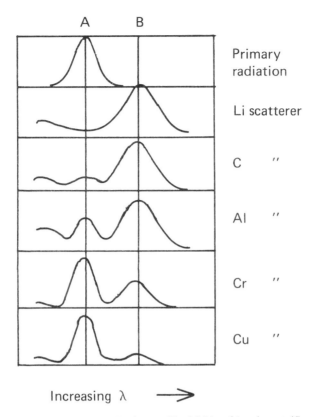

Fig. 1.14 The relative intensity of coherent (Rayleigh) and incoherent (Compton) scattering for different elements. Peaks A and B are coherent and incoherent respectively. (After Woo, 1926)

The expression in (1.44) has to be multiplied by the square of a *form factor* (or *atomic structure factor*) which takes account of the coherent scattering from all parts of the atom, and which is a function of the scattering angle and the wavelength of the radiation. The form factor approaches Z for small angles and long wavelengths, and falls with increasing angle. The angular distribution of the coherently scattered radiation thus becomes more peaked in the forward direction.

We may therefore expect the coherent part of the scattered radiation to be strongest in the heavier elements, as illustrated in Fig. 1.14. Its contribution to the removal of radiation from a parallel beam is, however usually small, mainly because of the very high photoelectric cross section in heavy elements. But at photon energies just below the absorption discontinuities it may become appreciable, as shown in Fig. 1.15. There is a small region of the (E_γ, Z) domain in which the contribution exceeds 20%.

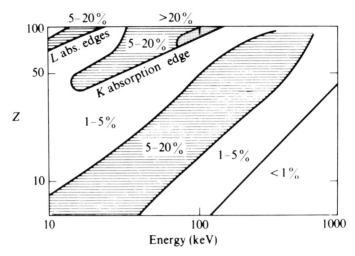

Fig. 1.15   Relative importance of coherent (Rayleigh) scattering compared with the total interaction cross-section from all processes (Dyson, 1973)

The extension of the theory of Thomson scattering to many-electron atoms is termed *Rayleigh scattering*, and is of fundamental importance in x-ray diffraction by crystals. When Rayleigh scattering occurs coherently from large numbers of atoms in a crystal, it produces the 'Bragg peak' in a crystal diffracto-meter, and also the discrete reflections in diffraction photographs. It goes beyond the scope of the present work to discuss these and other topics relating to the diffraction of x-rays and γ-rays by periodic structures; the basic interactions described in this chapter are however sufficient to give a good understanding of the behaviour of radiation in the context of the applications described in this book. The several processes discussed so far, and two further processes still to be described are combined together in the cross-section diagram in Fig. 1.16.

1.11 PAIR PRODUCTION

The processes discussed so far have depended upon either the 'quantum' behaviour of a photon (possessing energy and momentum) interacting with matter (Photo-electric, Compton processes) or the 'classical' behaviour of electromagnetic radiation setting charges into periodic motion (Thomson, Rayleigh processes). If the photon energy exceeds a certain value, other processes become possible. The conversion of electromagnetic radiation into matter is such a process. When the energy of the photon exceeds $2\, m_0 c^2$ (1.022 MeV), where m_0 is the rest-mass of the electron, it is possible, in principle, for a positron–electron pair to be formed, each particle carrying off any excess of energy as kinetic energy. It is necessary for *two* particles to be emitted in order to conserve charge, so no processes of this type are observed below this threshold energy.

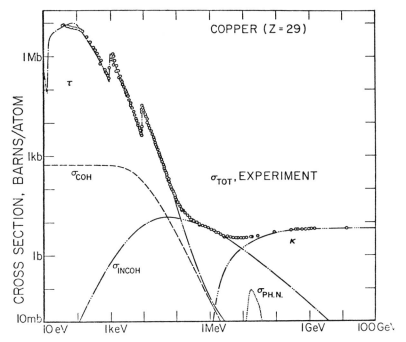

Fig. 1.16 γ-ray attenuation processes for copper (Hubbell, 1970)

If this process is examined for conservation of momentum, we see that the total momentum for the two charged particles cannot exceed

$$\frac{1}{c}\{(U_+^2 - m^2c^4)^{1/2} + (U_-^2 - m^2c^4)^{1/2}\}, \qquad (1.45)$$

and is in fact equal to this in the limiting case, in which both particles are propagated in the same direction from the point of production.

By inspection we see that this combined maximum momentum is always less than the momentum p_γ of the initial γ-ray photon, which is $\frac{1}{c}(U_+ + U_-)$.

To conserve momentum therefore, an additional body must be present. This can be supplied by a nucleus, and the interaction with it takes place *via* its Coulomb field. The cross-section for the process would therefore be expected to rise. with atomic number. More detailed considerations, which have been verified by experiment, show that the cross-section is proportional to Z^2. The process becomes more probable as E_γ increases (because the difference between expression (1.45) and p_γ becomes progressively less).

The momentum can be divided between positron and electron in any proportion, but the most probable events are those in which the momentum is divided equally, essentially because this maximises the momentum given by (1.45), thereby minimising the momentum which has to be taken up by the nucleus. The total cross-section (that is integrated over all energies and directions of the emergent particles) is included in the data for copper illustrated in Fig. 1.16. Clearly pair production becomes important at high γ-ray energies and would be even more important at high atomic numbers.

The relative importance of the three absorption processes discussed so far is best illustrated by the diagram in Fig. 1.17. This shows the regions of Z and E_γ where each process predominates.

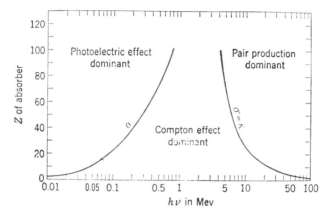

Fig. 1.17   Relative importance of photoelectric absorption, Compton scattering and pair production (Evans, 1955)

1.12 PROCESSES INVOLVING NUCLEAR ENERGY LEVELS

Because of the existence of the Coulomb field around the nucleus, it is possible, in principle, for γ-ray photons to interact with it, raising the nucleus to an excited state. These states have a mean-life given by $1/p$, where p is the probability per unit time of decay to a state of lower energy or to the ground state. The states therefore have a definite width, Γ, related to the mean life through the uncertainty principle,

$$\tau_m \Gamma = \hbar \qquad (1.46)$$

Their probability per unit time of decay is given by $\dfrac{1}{\tau_m}$ or $\Gamma/\hbar$. We are therefore dealing with a resonant process, and the cross-section (expressed as a function of E_γ, the incident photon energy) is given by the 'Lorenz' expression for resonance

$$\sigma \propto \frac{\Gamma^2}{(E - E_\gamma)^2 + \Gamma^2/4}. \qquad (1.47)$$

To find the constant of proportionality, more detailed considerations are necessary:

First, if the level can decay by more than one mode, we represent these by probabilities per unit time $(p_1, p_2, p_3,$ etc.) giving rise to *partial widths* $\hbar p_1, \hbar p_2, \hbar p_3 \ldots$, written as $\Gamma_1, \Gamma_2, \Gamma_3$ etc. In the present context, we identify Γ_γ and Γ_e as the *partial widths* for gamma emission and its frequently-encountered alternative, internal conversion. The fraction of excited nuclei decaying by γ-emission will be Γ_γ/Γ, and a detailed consideration shows that the cross-section for excitation by γ-radiation is reduced by the same factor. Secondly, the cross-section at resonance can be shown to be of the order of $\lambdabar^2$, and is given quantitatively by $4\pi\lambdabar^2$ (where $\lambdabar^2$ is the reduced wavelength, $\lambda/2\pi$) or λ^2/π. Thirdly, the cross section has to be multiplied by a statistical factor g, given by

$$g = \tfrac{1}{2}\frac{2I_e + 1}{2I_g + 1} \tag{1.48}$$

where $2I_e + 1$ and $2I_g + 1$ are the multiplicities of the excited and ground states respectively, and the factor of $\tfrac{1}{2}$ takes account of the fact that the incident photon has 2 possible states of polarisation. Therefore we may write

$$\sigma(E) = \frac{\lambda^2}{4\pi} g \frac{\Gamma^2}{(E - E_\gamma)^2 + (\Gamma/2)^2} \frac{\Gamma_\gamma}{\Gamma} \tag{1.49}$$

which is essentially the Breit–Wigner relation, derived originally for slow-neutron resonances as discussed in this book in section 2.2. (See also Appendix 4.)

We see therefore that nuclear resonant absorption is accompanied by nuclear resonance fluorescence or scattering, these terms tending to be used interchangeably in this context.

The lifetimes of nuclear excited states tend to lie in the range 10^{-8} s–10^{-14} s, corresponding to widths of 1 eV or less. A life-time of 10^{-8} seconds corresponds to a width of only 10^{-7} eV. Evidently these resonances will be greatly *broadened* by the Doppler effect produced by motion of source and absorber. They will also be *displaced* because of the energy of recoil of the γ-emitting nucleus and because of the corresponding effect of the absorbing nucleus. (that is the absorbing nucleus must recoil in order to take up the momentum of the incoming photon). Both these energies of recoil are given by

$$E_{\text{rec.}} = \frac{E_\gamma^2}{2Mc^2} \tag{1.50}$$

where M is the nuclear mass.

The line profiles for emission and absorption therefore appear somewhat as in Fig. 1.18, from which it may be seen that observation of the effect depends upon the overlap between the two profiles.

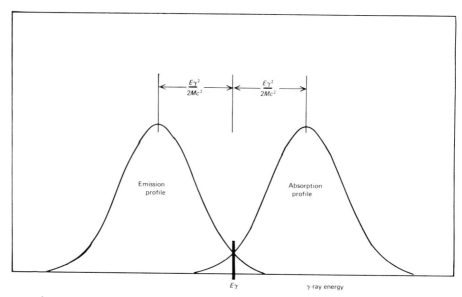

Fig. 1.18 Emission and Absorption profiles for nuclear resonant scattering, in conditions of Doppler broadening

Evidently the cross-section for nuclear resonant absorption is normally much less than given by (1.49), and, in general, it is small in comparison with the other processes discussed in this chapter.

The process is best observed in a scattering (rather than an absorption) experiment, and requires a method of experimentally controlling the degree of overlap shown in Fig. 1.18. This may be achieved by fast mechanical motion of the source, by altering the temperature of source or absorber, by making use of recoil caused by some preceding event, for example the emission of a β-particle or neutrino in radioactive decay, or by utilizing the motion caused by the 'Coulomb Fragmentation' of molecules in which an atom decays by electron capture – the subsequent loss of Auger electrons causes the emitting atom to acquire a positive charge which may, when distributed throughout the molecule, generate Coulomb forces which are sufficient to break up the molecule, causing the atoms to fly apart with velocities which may be considerable.

Nuclear resonant scattering has been applied to practical situations in radiation physics. A recent example of such an application has been reported by Vartsky *et al.* (1979), whose paper also includes theoretical analysis and references to previously-reported applications. Their particular study has been to determine iron levels in the human liver. They use a gaseous source of $^{56}MnCl_2$

to excite resonance in the ^{56}Fe in the liver iron stores, detecting the resonantly-scattered radiation (847 keV) by means of a Ge(Li) detector. The effective width of the γ-ray line is of the order of 1 eV, and overlap is ensured by making use of the recoil from the previously-emitted β-particle. Although the source has to be heated to over 1000°C, technical problems have been overcome and the method has been found feasible for the *in vivo* measurement of normal and elevated iron levels.

At higher γ-ray energies, reactions involving particle emission (for example $(γ,n)$, $(γ,2n)$) become possible. These photodisintegration reactions tend to produce a maximum cross-section in the region of 15–20 MeV, which is in the shape of a broad resonance, known as a *giant resonance*. Collective motion of the nucleons occurs, and the example illustrated in Fig. 1.19 is an electric dipole resonance. This type of interaction makes a contribution to the removal of photons from a beam, but its importance in a practical situation lies in the fact that neutrons are released. The possible appearance of neutrons in γ-ray shielding is a problem which has to be taken note of, as a factor influencing the design of shielding systems.

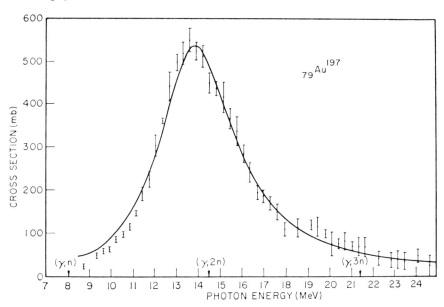

Fig. 1.19 Photonuclear absorption cross-section (Giant dipole resonance) in ^{197}Au (Fultz *et al.* 1962)

FURTHER READING

Burcham, W. E. (1979) *Elements of Nuclear Physics* Longman
Cohen, B. L. (1971) *Concepts of Nuclear Physics* Tata McGraw-Hill

Evans, R. D. (1955) *The atomic nucleus* McGraw-Hill
Mladjenović, M. (1973) *Radioisotope and radiation physics* Academic Press
Segrè, E. (1977) *Nuclei and Particles* Benjamin

REFERENCES

Dyson N. A. (1973) *X-rays in atomic and nuclear physics* Longman
Eddy, C. E. (1929) *Proc. Camb. Phil. Soc.,* **25**, 50
Fultz, S. C., Bramblett, R. L., Caldwell, J. T. and Kerr, N. A. (1962) *Phys. Rev.,* **127**, 1273
Hubbell, J. H. (1970) *Physics Bull.,* **21**, 353
James, R. W. (1967) *The optical principles of the diffraction of X-rays* Bell
Katz, L. and Penfold, A. S. (1952), *Revs. Mod. Phys.,* **24**, 28
Seliger, H. H. (1955) *Phys. Rev.,* **100**, 1029
Vartsky, D., Ellis, K. J., Hull, D. M. and Cohn, S. H. (1979) *Phys. Med. Biol.,* **24**, 689
Williamson, C. F., Boujet, J.-P. and Picard, J. (1966) Report CEA-R 3042 Centre d'Etudes Nucleaires de Saclay
Woo, Y. H. (1926) *Phys. Rev.,* **27**, 119

CHAPTER 2

Nuclear reactions and the production of radioisotopes

2.1 INTRODUCTION: NUCLEAR STABILITY

The behaviour of a nucleus under bombardment by neutrons or charged particles is strongly influenced by its binding energy. Because the binding energy is a measure of the stability of a nucleus, the stability, or otherwise, of a nucleus depends on its binding energy in relation to that of other nuclei of similar mass. A nucleus is held together by the 'strong interaction' between nucleons, which is offset to some extent by the Coulomb repulsion between protons. The study of the internal organisation of a nucleus is therefore one of the central aims of nuclear structure physics. The form of the variation of average binding energy per nucleon is shown in Fig. 2.1, from which it can be seen that for a wide

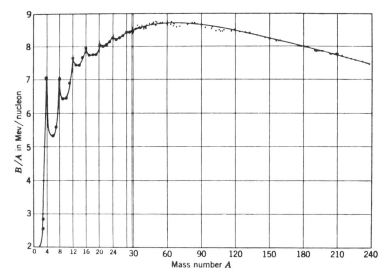

Fig. 2.1 Binding energy per nucleon. The peaks in binding energy, when A is a multiple of four, should be noted (Evans, 1955)

range of values of mass number this quantity is in the region of 8 MeV, declining to lower values for low and high A.

Certain light nuclei, notably those in which the nucleons are associated in groups of 4 or multiples of 4, have a relatively high degree of stability compared with their immediate neighbours. There are also other, smaller, peaks in certain regions of higher mass numbers, corresponding to shell closure for values of Z or $N = 20, 28, 50, 82, 126$, which are so-called 'magic numbers' predicted by the nuclear shell model (Cohen, 1971; Segrè, 1977).

The 'semi-empirical mass formula' (Appendix 3) is built up from a number of terms each representing a mass–energy contribution derived from simple assumptions regarding the forces between nucleons. These forces are supposed to be 'saturated', that is to say, the force between two nucleons is not affected by the proximity of other nucleons, and they resemble the forces between molecules in a liquid drop. Nucleons near the surface are less strongly bound, giving rise to the second term in the square brackets of (A 3.2). Coulomb repulsion is represented by an electrostatic term, and the fourth term represents the 'symmetry energy' of the nucleus, being zero where $N = Z$. The presence of nucleons with unpaired spins (that is due to Z or N (or both) being odd) requires the inclusion of a fifth term, known as the 'pairing energy'. The complete expression is shown in (A 3.2). The variation of mass–energy with Z, for a given A, determines the mechanism of radioactive decay, which is discussed in Chapter 4. The achievement of nuclear stability consists in minimising this mass–energy by successive decay processes. The semi-empirical mass formula is treated in detail in the nuclear physics texts already cited.

If the stable isotopes are plotted on a (Z, N) diagram, as shown in Fig. 2.2, they are seen to cluster about a 'line of stability' which, for lighter atoms, corresponds to $Z = N$. As the atomic mass number is increased, the stable isotopes depart systematically from this line. This is because the increasing number of protons causes an increased Coulomb repulsion, which has to be balanced by increasing the numbers of neutrons relative to protons. In this way, stability is maintained up to the point at which it becomes energetically favourable for an α-particle to be emitted. α-decay becomes common for $A > 206$.

The (Z, N) diagram is used as a basis for the widely-used Segrè Chart in which each nuclide is allocated a space in which we can summarise its nuclear properties, and on which the relationships between adjoining nuclides can be seen clearly. A small part of such a chart is shown in Fig. 2.3.

The manner in which the mass-energy varies with Z, for a given mass-number, is illustrated in Fig. 2.4. In the case of nuclei with a mass-number which is odd (that is, which consist of an odd number of one type of nucleon and an even number of the other), all nuclei of a given A lie on a single curve, parabolic in shape, as shown in Fig. 2.4(a). If the mass-number is even, two curves are required, one for 'odd–odd' and the other for 'even–even' nuclei (Fig. 2.4(b)). The even–even nuclides have a somewhat lower mass-energy than the odd–odd

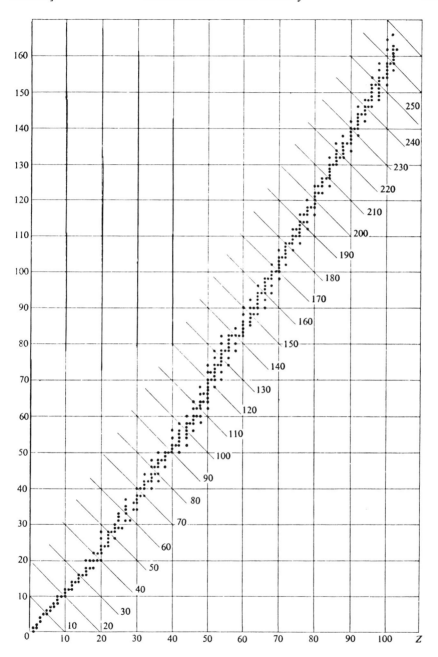

Fig 2.2 (Z,N) diagram for naturally occurring isotopes (Segrè, 1977)

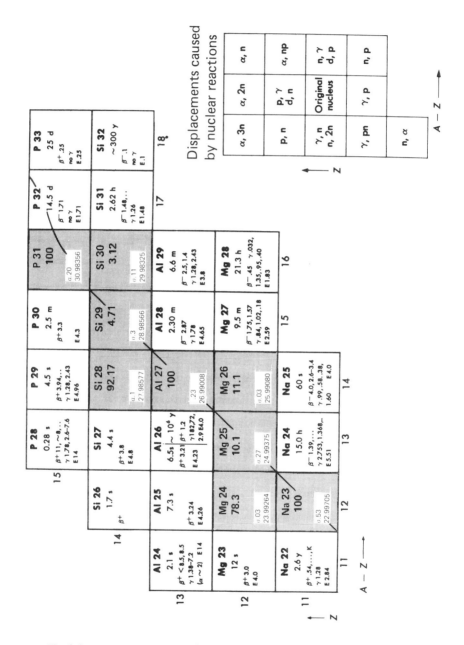

Fig. 2.3   A small part of a Segrè chart (Kaplan, 1962). The displacements caused by various nuclear reactions are also shown

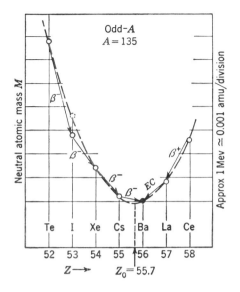

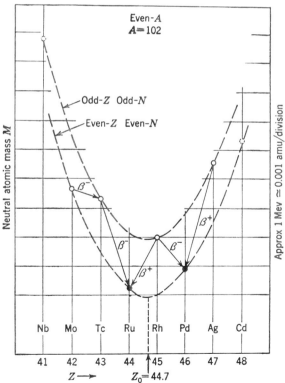

Fig. 2.4 Energy parabolae for $A = 135$ and $A = 102$ (Evans, 1955)

nuclides, because of the effect of the pairing-energy term, as outlined in Appendix 4. In the treatment of β-decay (section 4.2) it is shown that the mass-energy of the whole atom, and not that of the nucleus alone, is the relevant parameter. Accordingly this is the quantity plotted in Fig. 2.4.

The study of nuclear reactions involves an examination of the processes which take place when a neutron, proton, or other projectile approaches a nucleus with sufficient energy to overcome (in the case of charged particles) the Coulomb force of repulsion, and to come within range of the nuclear forces or, as they are known, the strong interaction. The projectile will then enter the nucleus, bringing not only its kinetic energy but also its binding energy. The subsequent behaviour of the system, which will involve the emission of gamma radiation or nucleons (or both) determines the nature of the products of the nuclear reaction. These products may or may not be radioactive; in the present context we shall naturally wish to emphasise the former alternative.

2.2 NEUTRON AND PROTON CAPTURE

The need to overcome Coulomb repulsion when a proton or α-particle is used as a projectile means that, except in the case of the lighter target nuclei, energies of several MeV are needed to cause a nuclear reaction to take place with measureable probability.

The absence of Coulomb forces when a neutron approaches a nucleus will place no lower limit on the kinetic energy of the incident particle, and hence we can examine nuclear reactions in their simplest form. The capture of a neutron (see Fig. 2.1) introduces 6–8 MeV of energy into the nucleus, and the energy levels of nuclei at this energy above the ground state are normally still discrete, although very close together (Fig. 2.5). Capture therefore depends upon the energy being of the correct amount needed to enable the product nucleus to be formed in one of its excited states, and is thus essentially resonant in nature. The cross-section for neutron capture is thus given by the 'Breit–Wigner' formula which, in its simplest form, may be written

$$\sigma = \pi \lambda^2 \frac{\Gamma^2}{(E - E_0)^2 + \Gamma^2/4} \tag{2.1}$$

where Γ is the width of the excited state and λ the reduced wavelength of the neutron.

De-excitation may take place by the emission of particles or gamma rays. Proton emission is less likely to occur because of the need to overcome the Coulomb barrier during exit, and neutron re-emission leaves the nucleus unchanged. The most significant process for us is therefore the emission of γ-radiation, with a probability given by the ratio of the 'radiative width' Γ_γ

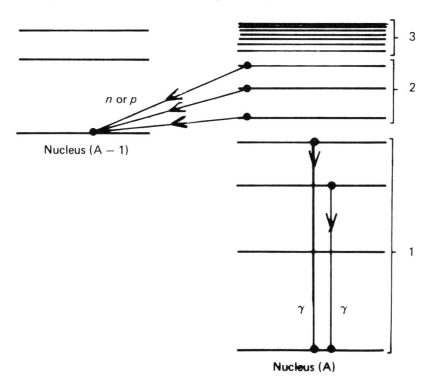

Fig. 2.5 Nuclear levels, illustrating the approach to the continuum. Region 1: Narrow levels excited by resonant absorption of γ-rays. Region 2: Broader levels from which the emission of a nucleon is possible, Region 3: very close overlapping levels forming a continuum

for this process, divided by the total width Γ. Hence the cross-section for the radiative capture, or (n,γ), process is given by

$$\sigma = \frac{\pi \lambdabar^2 \, \Gamma \Gamma_\gamma}{(E - E_0)^2 + \Gamma^2/4} \tag{2.2}$$

These resonances are superimposed on a slowly varying cross section which at low neutron energies may be shown (Appendix 4) to vary as $1/v$. Examples of this behaviour are showh in Fig. 2.6, and some further discussion of the Breit–Wigner formula is to be found in Appendix 4.

Using the neutron fluxes available in a nuclear reactor, radionuclides of high activity may be produced by the (n,γ) reaction. A few examples are given in Table 2.1. It will be apparent that radiative capture of neutrons will give rise to isotopes lying to the *left* of the line of stability shown in Fig. 2.2, and these will accordingly tend to decay by β^--decay. This will not always be so, because

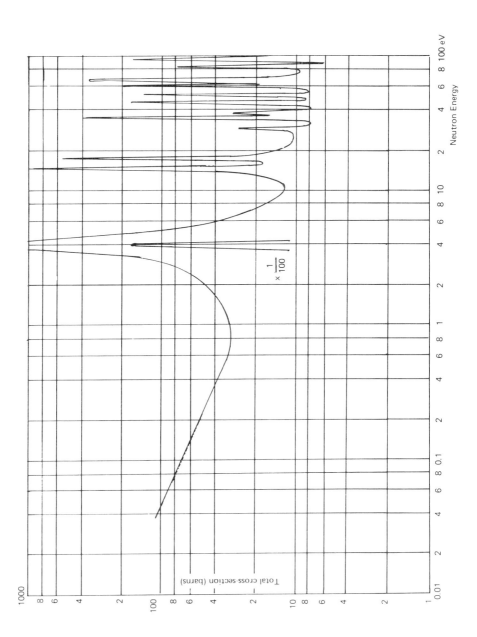

Fig. 2.6 Total neutron absorption cross-section for Thulium ($Z = 69$), illustrating
the 1/ v law (Appendix 4) and resonance (Hughes, 1958)

Table 2.1

Radiative capture cross-sections for (n,γ) reactions with thermal neutrons†

	σ_A	σ_B
$^{23}Na(n,\gamma)^{24}Na$	0.54	0.54
$^{27}Al(n,\gamma)^{28}Al$	0.21	0.21
$^{31}P(n,\gamma)^{32}P$	0.19	0.19
$^{40}A(n,\gamma)^{41}A$	0.53	0.53
$^{44}Ca(n,\gamma)^{45}Ca$	0.63	0.014
$^{59}Co(n,\gamma)^{60}Co$	37	37
$^{75}As(n,\gamma)^{76}As$	4.1	4.1
$^{81}Br(n,\gamma)^{82}Br$	2.6	1.6
$^{121}Sb(n,\gamma)^{122}Sb$	5.7	3.9
$^{123}Sb(n,\gamma)^{124}Sb$	3.9	1.07
$^{132}Ba(n,\gamma)^{133}Ba$	7	0.007
$^{191}Ir(n,\gamma)^{192}Ir$	960	370
$^{197}Au(n,\gamma)^{198}Au$	99	99

† Mean neutron velocity 2200 ms^{-1}.

σ_A: Radiative capture cross-section for the reaction in the pure isotope (Groshev *et al.* 1959).

σ_B: Effective activation (radiative capture) cross-section for the named isotope in a sample of the chemical element containing the isotope in its natural abundance (*The Radiochemical Manual*, 1966)

of the occurrence of certain odd-odd radionuclides which can decay by either β^- or β^+ decay (Fig. 2.4b), but it is a useful general rule.

The emission of a proton is of importance in certain reactions, for example in the reaction $^{14}N(n,p)^{14}C$, which is extensively used for the production of ^{14}C. Incidentally, this reaction is also responsible for the presence of this radionuclide in the atmosphere, as a result of the neutrons produced by cosmic-rays. The emission of a proton is energetically possible because of the loosely-bound 'last' proton in ^{15}N, readily emitted, in spite of the potential barrier at the nuclear surface.

Proton capture followed by *radiative de-excitation*, known as the (p,γ) reaction, has been much studied in the light elements. An example is illustrated in Fig. 2.7 showing the rich variety of resonances which occur in the excited nucleus ^{28}Si, following proton bombardment of aluminium.

2.3 COMPOUND NUCLEUS FORMATION

If there is much surplus energy, the highly-excited nucleus will enter a continuum of excited states. The resonant nature of the capture process is then not always apparent (Fig. 2.5). The emission of charged particles or neutrons by the nucleus becomes possible, though not before the nucleus has had time to distribute the incoming energy amongst several nucleons. Such a nucleus is termed a *compound*

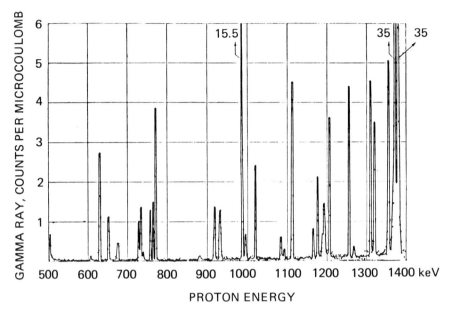

Fig. 2.7   Proton capture resonances in the ^{27}Al $(p,\gamma)^{28}$Si reaction (Brostrom *et al.*, 1947)

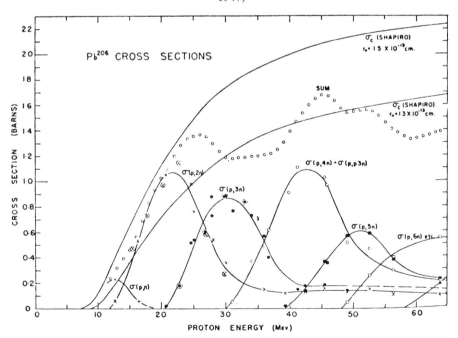

Fig. 2.8 (p,xn) excitation functions for proton bombardment of ^{206}Pb (Bell and Skarsgard, 1956)

nucleus, and the great majority of radioisotopes produced by charged particle bombardment are produced in this way by compound nucleus formation.

As the energy of the bombarding particles is increased, the emission of two or more nucleons may be more probable than the emission of one only. The several reactions shown in Fig. 2.8 are thus mutually competitive, and they add up to the cross-section for compound nucleus formation (shown by the heavy line) which rises, as the Coulomb repulsion is gradually overcome, to a limiting value approximately equal to the geometrical size of the nucleus.

The cross-section for a particular reaction is thus seen as a 'geometrical' cross-section multiplied by a probability factor which depends upon the relative probabilities of the several 'exit channels'.

Various exit channels are available to a compound nucleus and, of these alternatives, the emission of neutrons is more likely because of the inhibition of proton evaporation by Coulomb barrier effects.

It is an essential feature of the compound nucleus hypothesis that the possible methods of de-excitation are independent of the mode of formation of the compound nucleus. This is illustrated in Fig. 2.9 where the compound nucleus

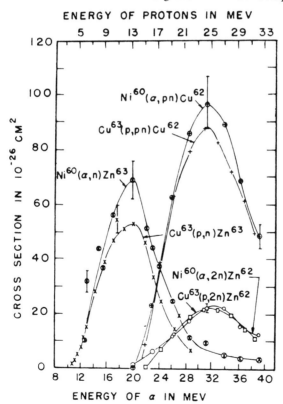

Fig. 2.9 Nuclear reactions taking place by two different routes (^{60}Ni + α and ^{63}Cu + p). In all cases the compound nucleus formed is ^{64}Zn (Ghoshal, 1950).

^{64}Zn is formed by two routes, ^{63}Cu $+ p$ and ^{60}Ni $+ \alpha$. The excitation functions of the ^{63}Cu$(p, n)^{63}$Zn and ^{60}Ni$(\alpha, n)^{63}$Zn reactions, and of other equivalent pairs, are the same in each case, once the energy scales have been normalised to take account of the different binding energies of the incident particles in the two cases.

2.4 DIRECT INTERACTION

The sharing of kinetic energy amongst the nucleons in a compound nucleus will be more likely to occur in nuclei consisting of many nucleons. In light nuclei, however, there is a significant chance that the incoming projectile will eject the nucleon with which it has just collided. No sharing of energy will take place. This process is called *direct interaction*, and can be identified experimentally by a study of the energy spectrum and angular distribution of the emergent nucleon. Clearly the energy of the ejected nucleon may be as high as the energy of an incident proton if the collision is essentially a two-nucleon event, in which case the energy spectrum will differ substantially from the evaporation spectra observed from compound nuclei.

When nuclear reactions occur by the mechanism of direct interaction the variation of cross-section with energy will not follow the pattern of the excitation functions as shown in Fig. 2.8. This aspect of the direct interaction process is an important factor in the production of radioisotopes. Furthermore, the ability of a fast neutron to eject a single fast proton, or *vice versa*, will be greater than would be the case if the reaction proceeded by compound nucleus formation.

The reactions ^{14}N$(n, p)^{14}$C and ^{7}Li$(p, n)^{7}$Be take place essentially by the direct interaction mechanism. The excitation function for the ^{12}C$(p, pn)^{11}$C reaction is illustrated in Fig. 2.10.

The direct interaction mechanism is important as a method of producing beams of fast neutrons for use in, for example, radiotherapy. The ability to produce neutrons carrying virtually the whole of the kinetic energy of an incident proton, as in the ^{7}Li$(p, n)^{7}$Be reaction, makes possible the production of a beam of relatively good penetrating power. Direct interaction plays a part in the production of neutrons by the deuteron bombardment of beryllium, ^{9}Be$(d, n)^{10}$B. It should be realised, however, that the additional possibility of 'stripping', in which the proton interacts with the beryllium nucleus and hence allows the neutron to continue in the forward direction, also makes a contribution to the fast neutron flux produced by this reaction. The production of neutrons by nuclear reactions is discussed in Chapter 6.

2.5 FISSION

A careful examination of the binding energy curve of Fig. 2.1 will show that it may be energetically favourable for a very heavy nucleus to divide into two components of approximately equal mass, which will occupy positions in the central part of the curve, where binding energies are at their greatest. A potential barrier has to be overcome before fission can occur, and the energy necessary for this may be obtained by the capture of a neutron. In the three nuclides ^{233}U, ^{235}U, ^{239}Pu, the binding energy alone of this neutron is sufficient to overcome the 'fission potential barrier', and the (n, f) process may thus occur by means of neutrons of thermal energy. Many other nuclei will undergo fission under fast neutron bombardment (for example ^{238}U, requiring a threshold energy of

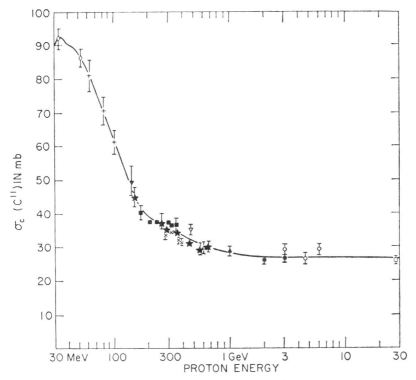

Fig. 2.10 Excitation function for a reaction proceeding by the direct interaction process (^{12}C$(p,pn)^{11}$C) (Cumming, 1963)   (© 1963 by Annual Reviews Inc.)

1 MeV). Several transuranic nuclei are spontaneously fissile, occasionally with probabilities sufficiently large in relation to other processes to lead to their being useful as laboratory sources of fission neutrons (for example, ^{244}Cm, ^{252}Cf). The probability of the latter process may be predicted from the semi-empirical mass formula (Appendix 3). The important parameter is shown to be the quantity Z^2/A. Spontaneous fission becomes more probable, that is, the half life for the process becomes progressively less, as this parameter increases. This is illustrated in Fig. 2.11.

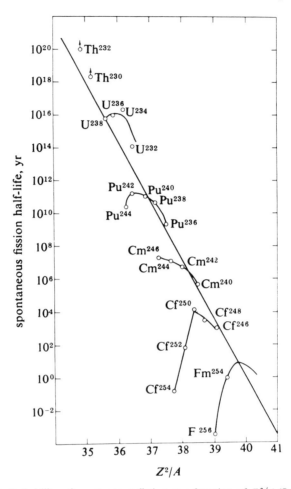

Fig. 2.11 Probability of spontaneous fission as a function of Z^2/A (Segrè, 1977)

When fission occurs, two or three neutrons are released, and these may induce further fissions, leading to a nuclear chain reaction which, when limited by the presence of neutron-absorbing materials, is the principle on which the nuclear reactor is based. Examination of Fig. 2.1 shows that energy of the order of 1 MeV per nucleon now becomes available. In fact, about 190 MeV is released in each fission process, of which ~170 MeV is available as kinetic energy of fission fragments. The remainder is lost from the system in the form of neutrinos or electromagnetic radiation. This energy release makes possible the production of power on a large scale in nuclear reactors.

The two fission fragments contain numbers of neutrons considerably in excess of those required for stability, that is they lie to the left of the 'line of stability' shown in Fig. 2.2. They therefore decay by β^--emission, and thus it can be seen that the fission process provides an important mechanism for the production of β^--emitters. The short-lived products, lying far from the line of stability, decay into longer-lived nuclides before achieving stability. The behaviour of these decay chains is represented by the equations developed in Appendix 5.

The neutron capture process explained in section 2.2 takes place readily in nuclear reactors. It should be added that there is also the possibility that the capture of several neutrons in sequence will produce a further range of neutron-rich products. If neutron capture alternates with β^--decay, the 'nucleosynthesis' of elements becomes possible. This is the main process by which the elements were formed in the early evolution of the universe, and by which process the transuranic elements ($92 < Z < 100$) may now be produced artificially. The process occurs slowly in nuclear reactors, but it has been found to produce a rich variety of transuranic elements in the extremely high neutron fluxes ($>10^{19}$ n cm^{-2} sec^{-1}) which occur near the centre of underground nuclear explosions.

Fission thus produces many β^--emitters. It should be mentioned that, in a few cases, the isotopes produced directly as a result of the fission process are so far from the line of stability, that is, so far along the *left* of the parabolic curves in Fig. 2.4, that the energy available for radioactive decay is sufficiently high for particle emission, in particular neutron emission, to be possible. This is observed for example in the fission products ^{137}I ($t_{1/2} = 23s$) and ^{87}Br ($t_{1/2} = 55s$). These 'delayed' neutrons appear with characteristic half-lives after the fission process (≈ 0.2–56 seconds for the main groups). They substantially lengthen the time constant for the neutron multiplication process in a reactor, so allowing the system to be effectively controlled.

2.6 SPALLATION AND HEAVY ION BOMBARDMENT

At higher bombarding energies, processes of a somewhat different nature may take place. If the energy of the incident particle exceeds about 50 MeV, many nucleons or small groups of nucleons may be ejected from the target nucleus. This can occur without the formation of a compound nucleus. At still higher energies (>150 MeV) the process probably occurrs at the nuclear surface, from which nuclear material may be dislodged. These processes, which are termed 'spallation', can produce reaction products differing by several units of Z from the target nucleus. A measurable yield of ^{38}Cl is produced for example, by bombarding copper with 70 MeV protons. The remaining nucleons are unlikely to combine to form just one nucleus, although Morrison (1953) has pointed out that on purely energetic grounds, the reaction ^{63}Cu$(p, n\,^{25}$Al$)^{38}$Cl is the most favourable of the many possible reactions leading to this particular product. The production of large numbers of individual nucleons is equally unlikely, on energetic grounds. It is evident that spallation, at least at moderate particle energies, proceeds by the emission of α-particles and other light nuclei (for example ^{8}Li) which have relatively high binding energies.

At even higher energies than this, say 500 MeV and above, fission is frequently observed, along with complete fragmentation of the nucleus, which reaction again produces a wide range of reaction products.

A further class of nuclear reactions occur when heavy ions, for example ^{12}C, ^{16}O, are used as projectiles. At low energies, Coulomb forces operate and Rutherford scattering is observed. Coulomb excitation of the nuclei can occur. At higher energies the two ions may come into contact, and transfer of nuclear matter takes place during reactions of the type ^{32}S(^{14}N,^{13}N)^{33}S. The transfer of single nucleons or small numbers of nucleons will not yield products differing in nature from those which result from more conventional processes. Transfer of larger numbers of nucleons does produce many reaction products well away from the line of stability, and this is a method of producing very short-lived isotopes not capable of being made by other processes.

If fusion of the projectile and its nucleus target occurs, the range of products is further extended. Many transuranic nuclides have been produced in this way.

2.7 QUANTITATIVE ASPECTS OF RADIOISOTOPE PRODUCTION

2.7.1 Charged particle bombardment by accelerator-produced beams

In all practical circumstances the proportion of bombarded atoms transmuted by the beam is small, and therefore we can assume that the number of target atoms remains constant, with negligible error.

Consider the case of steady charged-particle bombardment followed by decay. We assume that a thin target of uniform thickness is used, bombarded normally to its surface.

Let a = number of target atoms per unit target volume
g = target thickness
σ = reaction cross-section
λ = decay constant of radioactive product
n = number of radioactive atoms at time t during bombardment
N = number of incident particles per unit time
Therefore we may write

$$\mathrm{d}n = (N\sigma ag - n\lambda)\mathrm{d}t \qquad (2.3)$$

If the assumption is made that $n = 0$ at $t = 0$, it follows that

$$n = \frac{N\sigma ag}{\lambda}(1 - \mathrm{e}^{-\lambda t}) \qquad (2.4)$$

or the activity,

$$n\lambda = N\sigma ag\,(1 - e^{-\lambda t}). \tag{2.5}$$

If we introduce $\dfrac{N}{S}$ = the particle flux, ϕ, where S is the area of the supposedly uniform beam, and $U = Sag$ the number of target atoms, we may write this as

$$n\lambda = \phi\sigma U(1 - e^{-\lambda t}). \tag{2.6}$$

The activity thus builds up to an equilibrium, at which the rate of production equals the rate of decay. Bombardment for 3 and 4 half-lives gives a good approach to the theoretical maximum. This is given simply as

flux × cross-section × number of atoms.

This is often written as

flux × macroscopic cross-section × target volume,   (2.7)

where the macroscopic cross-section $\Sigma = \sigma a$.

2.7.2 Reactor irradiation
In this case appreciable burn-up of target material can occur. Assuming, for the moment, negligible decay during irradiation, we can write

$$dn = \phi\sigma agS\,dt, \quad \text{where } a \text{ is now variable, with initial value } a_0.$$

Therefore, $dn = \phi\sigma(U_0 - n)dt$, where $a_0 gS = U_0$ (2.8)

Hence (if $n = 0$ at $t = 0$ as before)

$$n = U_0(1 - e^{-\phi\sigma t}) \tag{2.9}$$

or, $n\lambda = \lambda U_0(1 - e^{-\phi\sigma t})$ (2.10)

We now have an approach to a saturation activity which is equal to the decay constant × the number of target atoms initially present: complete conversion to the radionuclide is implied by this result, after sufficiently long irradiation times.

If no restriction is placed on the rate of decay, that is if decay can occur during the irradiation, we may write

$$dn = (\sigma\phi U - n\lambda)dt \tag{2.11}$$

where U = number of unconverted atoms, $U_0 e^{-\phi\sigma t}$.

Therefore, $dn = (\sigma\phi U_0 e^{-\phi\sigma t} - n\lambda)dt$ (2.12)

the solution of which may be shown to be

$$n = \frac{\phi\sigma U_0}{\lambda - \phi\sigma} (e^{-\phi\sigma t} - e^{-\lambda t}). \tag{2.13}$$

The activity $n\lambda$ at small values of t is given by

$$n\lambda = \lambda\phi\sigma U_0 t, \tag{2.14}$$

rising linearly with time.

Note that the full expression implies that the activity reaches a maximum at a time

$$t_m = \frac{\ln\phi\sigma - \ln\lambda}{\phi\sigma - \lambda}. \tag{2.15}$$

The value of the activity $n\lambda$ at this time is then given by

$$\lambda U_0 e^{-\lambda t_m} \tag{2.16}$$

Clearly the maximum activity occurs at an earlier time, and is itself greater, the higher the neutron flux.

A further limitation is imposed by burn-up of the *product* nucleus by additional neutron capture. Equation (2.11) now becomes

$$dn = [\sigma\phi U - n(\lambda + \sigma'\phi)]dt \tag{2.17}$$

and $$n = \frac{\phi\sigma U_0}{\lambda - \phi\sigma + \phi\sigma'} (e^{-\phi\sigma t} - e^{-(\lambda + \phi\sigma')t}) \tag{2.18}$$

where σ' is the neutron cross-section of the product nucleus.

It will be apparent that burn-up of the product nucleus in this manner will reduce the magnitude of the maximum activity and also the time at which it occurs.

A practical example of the use of these equations is given in section 2.8.

2.8 PRACTICAL ASPECTS OF RADIOISOTOPE PRODUCTION

The foregoing review of nuclear reactions will have given some indication of the principles to be followed when choosing a suitable reaction for the production of a given radionuclide. Neutron-rich isotopes are normally produced by neutron capture or by nuclear fission in a reactor. Neutron-deficient isotopes normally require charged-particle bombardment in an accelerator, for example a fixed frequency ('classical') cyclotron. Very many isotopes can be obtained commercially but some, particularly those with half-lives less than a few hours, may have to be produced locally, and this depends upon the availability of a suitable accelerator.

2.8.1 The target material
The form of the target material for reactor irradiation is determined mainly by the need to withstand a moderate temperature rise, which may be in the region of $100°$-$200°C$ in reactors used for radioisotope production. This is not a serious limitation, and allows the use of metallic samples in foil or powdered form, and a wide range of inorganic salts in the anhydrous state. The range of materials investigated by neutron activation analysis is even wider. The samples to be irradiated are normally sealed in small aluminium cans, and are subject to a temperature test before the can is placed in the reactor. After irradiation, followed by a waiting period to allow the short-lived products to decay, the container may be opened and the material chemically processed.

The physical dimensions of materials for reactor irradiation must be sufficiently small to ensure that the neutron flux is not significantly attenuated, because this would cause shielding of part of the target material. This requirement corresponds to the condition $\ell \ll \Sigma^{-1}$ where ℓ represents the linear dimensions of the target and Σ the mean macroscopic (total) cross-section for the neutron spectrum and target materials used. Linear dimensions of the order of a few centimeters are often permissible, but this would not be the case in the example quoted earlier ($^{59}Co(n, \gamma)^{60}Co$) where the mean cross-section (37 barn) and number of atoms per unit volume of cobalt metal ($\sim 10^{23}$ cm^{-3}) combine to give a macroscopic cross-section of 3.7 cm^{-1}, limiting the thickness of a disc to 2-3 mm only.

When a target is to be bombarded in a charged-particle beam, the thickness need be no greater than the range of the particles, normally much less than 1 mm. The target must, however, be designed to withstand much higher temperatures. In the internal beam of a cyclotron, a current of 100-$500\,\mu A$ at a particle energy of 10 MeV may be available, and the dissipation of several kilowatts of energy requires careful design of the target cooling system. A rotating target will reduce the surface temperatures attained, but the surface temperature will still normally be the factor limiting the current which can safely be used.

By designing the target so that the beam is at glancing incidence, the effective beam area is increased, thereby reducing the surface temperature. If the target material is a poor thermal conductor, it may be pressed into a water-cooled ribbed copper plate, and the thickness of the target material kept to the minimum value compatible with adequate yield of the desired radioisotopes.

If the external beam of a cyclotron is used, the target will be outside the machine vacuum, and the restrictions on target materials can be considerably relaxed. Non-metallic targets become practicable, for example crystalline NaBr for the production of ^{81}Rb used in ^{81}Kr generators (see section 2.8.5 below) or liquid targets for example, water for the production of ^{18}F by the ^{16}O(^{3}He,p)^{18}F reaction. Gaseous targets, in the form of gases flowing through an irradiation chamber, are also practicable.

2.8.2 Specific activity

The specific activity of a radioisotope is the *activity per unit mass* of the stable element present. For many 'tracer' applications the specific activity has to be as high as possible, so that the amount of stable material introduced for instance into a biological system or the human subject, is not sufficient to disturb the normal behaviour of the system. On the other hand, chemical processing in the total absence of stable 'carrier' is difficult because of the very small concentration (in chemical terms) of the radioactive substance, which is normally present only in sub-weighable quantities. A compromise therefore has to be sought.

In cases where (n,γ) reactions occur in reactor irradiations, the radioactive product is an isotope of the same element as the starting material. The radioisotope will therefore be inseparable by ordinary chemical means from the stable isotopes of that element, and this fact limits the specific activity which can be attained. Even so, activities of several curies per gram are frequently quoted, in practical handbooks of radioisotope production.

When the radioactive half-life is of the order of one year or more, it is sometimes possible for the proportion of atoms converted to be an appreciable fraction of the whole. However, the target material must not be left in the reactor for so long that a second neutron capture process takes place in the desired product atoms. A good example of this is the production of ^{60}Co by the ^{59}Co(n,γ)^{60}Co reaction. A significant fraction of ^{59}Co is converted to ^{60}Co after a few months irradiation in a high flux reactor but if the target material is left too long, ^{61}Co (decaying quickly to ^{61}Ni) may be produced in significant quantities. Nevertheless a 'saturation' activity of 900 Ci g^{-1} is possible, compared with the absolute theoretical maximum of about 1200 Ci g^{-1}.

In the case of fission products, specific activities are much higher than most (n,γ) products, although limited by the presence of stable isotopes of the same element, produced as end-products of one or other of the many decay chains which are possible, following fission. As an example, the maximum theoretical specific activity of ^{137}Cs is about 100 Ci g^{-1}, but is limited to about 25 Ci g^{-1} by the presence of stable ^{134}Cs in fission products.

2.8.3 Radionuclidic purity

This may be defined as the proportion of total activity which is in the desired, or specified, form. In a few cases, a radioisotope may be prepared by reactor irradiation and is then ready for use without any processing. Examples are ^{60}Co sources used for teletherapy, produced by neutron irradiation of metallic cobalt. Iridium–192 is much used for brachy therapy, in which the active material is placed in close proximity to the site being treated, and is prepared by reactor irradiation of iridium wire. Iron–55, which decays by electron capture emitting the characteristic x-rays of manganese, is prepared by reactor irradiation of separated isotope ^{54}Fe in the form of the oxide Fe_2O_3 and may then be used without processing, although it is normally distributed as an acidic solution of ferric chloride for convenience in dispensing. More usually, some form of separation is needed to ensure radionuclidic purity, which may then be checked by observing the decay as a function of time (to test for the presence of interfering half-lives), or by study of the γ-ray spectrum to look for impurity lines in the spectrum.

To minimise impurities consisting of other radioisotopes of the same element, attention must be paid to the nature of the irradiated material, and, in the case of cyclotron-bombarded targets, to the energy of the incident beam. Isotopically separated targets are used for both reactor and cyclotron irradiations when necessary, but in the case of cyclotron bombardment, reference to the excitation functions, as for example in Fig. 2.8, will usually suggest an optimum beam energy. When this is done, the choice of target thickness becomes an important consideration: by ensuring that the beam emerges from the far side of the target before being slowed down to too low an energy, the (α,n) or (p,n) reactions can be minimised relative to the $(\alpha,2n)$, $(\alpha,3n)$, and other reactions, which may be the processes desired. In such cases the target will often be a layer of material evaporated or sputtered on to a more massive target base, of good thermal conductivity. The excitation functions may be studied by bombarding a stack of foils of known individual thickness, and then observing the relative activities of different isotopes as a function of depth within the stack.

2.8.4 Preparation for medical or biological use

When the radioisotope is to be used for medical or biological work, either as a tracer in diagnostic tests or therapeutically, the question of its purity is of particular importance. So far as *radionuclidic* purity is concerned, the presence of additional radioisotopes of the same element will not necessarily invalidate tracer experiments carried out with the material, provided all measurements are made with reference to standards prepared from the same material. But in general the additional radioisotopes will have different half-lives from that of the specified radionuclide, leading to a decay curve which will no longer be a simple exponential, and to a spectrum of β- and γ- activity which changes with time. Furthermore, the presence of long-lived radioisotopic impurities may materially increase the radiation dose absorbed by the patient who is undergoing the diagnostic test. Radionuclidic purity is therefore clearly desirable in most applications.

Radiochemical purity is that proportion of the total activity which is in the specified chemical form. Clearly a high degree of radiochemical purity is desirable – for example, the presence of an appreciable amount of organic iodine, in a sample of inorganic iodide intended to be used for thyroid diagnostic measurements, would affect any measurements of percentage thyroid uptake.

Chemical purity must naturally be considered in any medical or biological application, although the amounts of stable chemical materials present, either as carriers or impurity, are usually so small that this is not normally a problem. This is because the radionuclide will normally have been prepared from materials of the highest available purity.

If the preparation is required for intravenous injection it will need to be free of pyrogens, which are organic products of bacterial activity causing a febrile reaction when injected, will also need to be bacteriologically sterile, and to be in a solution which is isotonic with respect to the intracellular fluids. Isotonic saline is normally used as the medium for the intravenous administration of radionuclides, but if the material is for oral administration this is not a necessary requirement.

2.8.5 Production from a 'generator'

If a radioisotope has a half-life which is inconveniently short for transportation from a distant production facility, it can sometimes be made, in the laboratory or clinic where it is to be used, by the decay of a radioactive parent of longer half-life. An example of this is ^{132}I (half-life 2.3h) which has been found to be of great value in thyroid diagnostic work (see section 5.5). It may be obtained by decay of the parent isotope ^{132}Te (half-life 78h) which is readily obtained by the fission of uranium:

$$\mathrm{U}(n,f) \longrightarrow {}^{132}\mathrm{Te} \xrightarrow[78\mathrm{h}]{\beta^-} {}^{132}\mathrm{I} \xrightarrow{\beta^-} {}^{132}\underline{\mathrm{Xe}} \text{ (stable)}$$

^{132}I activity therefore 'grows' in a ^{132}Te preparation, from zero to an equilibrium activity at which the rate of decay is equal to the rate of production. 1mCi of ^{132}Te will then thus have 1mCi of ^{132}I in equilibrium with it, if it has been allowed to stand undisturbed for several ^{132}I half-lives. This is a type of equilibrium observable in the case of certain naturally occurring radioelements (for example ^{226}Ra in equilibrium with ^{222}Rn), the parent and daughter activities then decaying slowly, with the half-life of the parent nuclide. We see from the 'growth' equation in Appendix 5 that one half of the daughter activity is generated after 1 half-life, three-quarters after 2 half-lives, etc., so that after 3 or 4 half-lives an amount can be 'milked' off which is almost equal to the activity of the parent. ^{132}Te is prepared in the form of a 'generator' of sodium tellurite adsorbed on a column of alumina, from which ^{132}I can be eluted using dilute ammonium hydroxide.

Another example of the use of a generator is for the supply of the radio-isotope ^{99m}Tc. This is used extensively for organ scanning and for imaging with gamma-cameras, because of the convenient γ-ray energy emitted (190 keV). It is prepared from ^{99}Mo, produced by the (n,γ) reaction on ^{98}Mo, or by uranium fission. The genetic relationships are best shown in the diagram:

$$^{98}\underline{Mo} \quad \xrightarrow[67h]{(n,\gamma)} \quad ^{99}Mo \quad \xrightarrow{90\%} \quad ^{99m}Tc \quad \xrightarrow[6\ hr]{I.T.} \quad ^{99}Tc \quad \left(\xrightarrow{2.2 \times 10^5 y} \quad ^{99}Ru \right)$$
$$\xrightarrow{10\%}$$

The ^{99}Mo is adsorbed on to a column as molybdate, from which the technicium can be eluted as pertechnetate.

The gaseous radioisotope ^{81}Kr referred to in section 2.8.1 is 'generated' from ^{81}Rb, produced by the bombardment of bromine in the form of sodium bromide, and the use of this isotope in lung function and in perfusion studies is increasing because of its availability in this form.

The principle of the generator thus makes available certain radionuclides which, in at least two instances, have become widely used, and whose short half-lives would otherwise have precluded this.

FURTHER READING

Eichholz, G. G. (Ed.) (1972) *'Radioisotope Engineering'* Dekker.
The Radiochemical Manual (1966) The Radiochemical Centre, Amersham.

REFERENCES

Bell, R. E. and Skarsgard, H. M. (1956) *Can. J. Phys.,* **34**, 745
Brostrom, K. J. and Huus, T. (1947) *Phys. Rev.,* **71**, 661
Cohen, B. L. (1971) See Further Reading for Chapter 1
Cumming, J. B. (1973) *Ann. Rev. Nucl. Sci.,* **13**, 261
Evans, R. D. (1955) See Further Reading for Chapter 1
Ghoshal, S. N. (1950) *Phys. Rev.,* **80**, 939
Groshev, L. V., Demidov, A. M., Lutsenko, U. N. and Pelekhov, V. I. (1959)
    Atlas of γ-ray spectra from radiative capture of thermal neutrons Pergamon
Hughes, D. J. and Schwartz, R. B. (1958) *Neutron cross-sections* Brookhaven
    National Laboratory Report BNL 325, and Supplements
Kaplan, I. (1962) *Nuclear Physics* Addison–Wesley
Segrè, E. (1977) See Further Reading for Chapter 1

Instrumentation – an introduction to α-, β-, and γ-radiation detectors

---

3.1 INTRODUCTORY

The detection of nuclear radiation is based on the several interactions between radiation and matter discussed in Chapter 1. Ionization processes are of paramount importance, and the ability of ionizing radiation to discharge an electroscope was one of the earliest observations to be made at the time of discovery of x-rays and of radioactivity. The principle involved is the ionization of a gas by α-, β-, or γ-radiation, and the separation of the charges thus produced, using an electrostatic field. The change in position of these charges, and their subsequent arrival at the electrodes produces changes of potential (if the electrodes are connected to a high voltage supply through a suitably large resistor) which may be converted into pulses and then amplified. Alternatively, the continuously collected charge may be measured directly as an ionization current. We expect therefore that a gas-filled tube containing two electrodes connected to a high voltage supply will be the basis of an important class of detectors. We shall see below that the Geiger and proportional counters, and also the ionization chamber, are all extensively used in applied nuclear and radiation physics.

We might note in passing that the ability of electromagnetic radiation to produce ionization by a direct process is limited to the release of single electrons (or, at most, an electron-positron pair) by the processes of the photoelectric effect, the Compton effect, and pair production. By far the greater amount of ionization in a gas-dector is produced, however, by the subsequent slowing down of these electrons. For this reason γ-radiation is sometimes known as 'indirectly-ionizing' radiation, because its detection depends essentially on the electrons released by this initial event.

Interactions with solids are attractive as a basis for radiation detection, because of the possibility of a much greater detection efficiency in comparison with gas detectors. The basic phenomena are, however, somewhat more complex. When an ionizing particle passes through a crystalline solid, excitation and ionization of optical levels of the material occurs, and the de-excitation may occur with the emission of visible light. If the crystal contains impurity atoms as 'activators', capture of an electron released in the ionization process may produce optical photons with increased probability. These optical photons may then be detected by means of a photomultiplier, producing a pulse which may then be amplified. This is the basis of the scintillation counter, which is widely used for the detection of γ-radiation. Many organic and plastic materials show luminescence when irradiated with ionizing radiation, and are extensively used for'β-particle detection.

Semiconductor materials are of great importance as radiation detectors. A system consisting of a $p-n$ junction operated under reverse-bias conditions has a suitably high resistance, and can detect charged particles entering its depletion layer. Because of the limited thickness of such 'barrier-layer' detectors, they are mainly used for the detection of α-particles, whose short range makes them very suitable for detection by this method.

If p-type semiconductor material is used, it may be compensated by drifting-in some donor atoms, such as lithium, under the influence of heat and an applied electric field. In this way, detectors with linear dimensions up to several centimetres can be fabricated, and these lithium-drifted silicon and germanium detectors are well-established in x-ray and nuclear physics, as tools for x-ray and γ-ray spectroscopy, and are appearing to an increasing extent in laboratories devoted to medical and radioisotope physics. The high-purity germanium detector is also coming into use, for γ-ray spectroscopy.

In the ensuing sections we shall discuss these various devices in turn, showing how they can be of use in the subject-areas covered by this book.

3.2 GEIGER AND PROPORTIONAL COUNTERS

The size of the voltage pulse produced by the passage of a single β-particle, followed by subsequent collection of all the ion-pairs, may be calculated if the number of ion-pairs and the electrical capacity between the two electrodes is known. The mean energy necessary to produce an ion-pair (denoted by W) is a quantity which has been carefully investigated, because of its importance in connection with radiation detector operation. Ionization of an atom can, in principle, take place from any electron shell, and it is also possible for atomic excitation to occur, which removes energy from the ionizing particle without producing an ion-pair. The relative weight which must be assigned to these processes cannot be calculated with any accuracy, and so main reliance must be placed on experimental studies. W is found to be approximately independent of the kinetic energy of the ionizing particles (electrons in the present context) but depends on the gas. The value for air has been particularly well-investigated because of the use of air-filled ionization chambers as the basis of ionization dosimetry (section 3.5), and the currently accepted value is 33.7 eV. A few values for other gases are given in Table 3.1, from which we see that the values lie mainly in the range 25–40 eV.

Table 3.1

Mean energy required to produce an ion-pair in
various gases (after Siegbahn, 1965)

	W_β eV	$W_\alpha(^{210}Po)$ eV
He	42.3	42.7
Ne	36.6	36.8
A	(26.4)	36.8
Kr	24.2	24.1
H_2	36.3	36.3
N_2	35.0	36.6
O_2	30.9	32.5
Air	33.7	

The number of ion-pairs produced by a particle of energy E, therefore, is E/W, and the size of the voltage pulse (assuming complete separation and collection of all the released charge) is given by

$$V = \frac{Ee}{C.W} \tag{3.1}$$

where C is the capacity of the ion chamber and e the electronic charge. By inserting typical values (for example $E = 10^5$ eV, $C = 10$ pF, $W = 30$ eV) we see that the pulse is very small (5×10^{-5} V in this example). Although such ion chambers can be used for the detection of individual events, the problems of electronic noise are such that their use is reserved for very energetic particles of short range, for example fission fragments, whose energies lie in the much higher range 60–100 MeV.

In order to produce a larger pulse from the β- or γ-radiation emitted in radioactive decay, use is made of the ability of an electron to create further ionizations by collision, if the electron is accelerated to a sufficient velocity between collisions. By successive collisions, each electron may release 2 or 3 further electrons, which are themselves accelerated sufficiently to produce further ionizations in turn. As many as 10^6 electrons may arrive at the positive electrode for every electron released by the original ionizing particle. This **Gas Multiplication** results in a large pulse appearing at the positive electrode, which can be used to actuate a recording device, such as a scaler, without electronic amplification. This is the principle of the Geiger counter. In order to achieve a field strength sufficiently high for the avalanching process to occur, it is normal to use a cylindrical geometry, with an outer cylinder and a wire along the axis, around which the required high field strength can be produced.

A Geiger counter, then, in its most typical form, consists of a metal cylinder (the cathode) 2–3 cm in diameter, normally earthed, and a concentric wire (the anode) connected to a positive potential of a few hundred volts. The connection is made through a high resistance so that when an avalanche occurs, as a result of an ionizing particle, the potential of the wire momentarily falls, and a negative-going pulse is provided at the anode terminal (Fig. 3.1). The counter is normally filled with argon or neon at a pressure somewhat below atmospheric pressure. An end-window is provided, with a thickness not exceeding 4 mg(cm)$^{-2}$, and this will admit the β-particles from a radioactive source, providing that their energy is greater than a certain value, which is in the region of 40 keV.

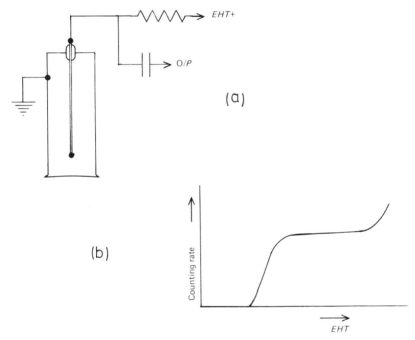

Fig. 3.1 (a) Geiger counter with its external connections. (b) Counting rate as a function of voltage applied to a Geiger counter showing the 'plateau' region

At low voltages, no gas multiplication will occur, but as the voltage is gradually increased, multiplication will commence, and eventually when an avalanche is triggered off by a β-particle, it will spread along the wire, involving its whole length. Any further increase of voltage will tend to promote a continuous discharge in the tube, and so the optimum voltage has to be found experimentally by recording the counting rate from a small β-emitting radioactive source placed near the window, as a function of applied voltage. The flat part of the curve (Fig. 3.1a) represents the working region of the counter's characteristic.

A β-particle entering the counter gas will be recorded with essentially 100% probability, but the overall sensitivity of the counter to the radiation from a given source is proportional to the fraction of β-particles managing to penetrate the window. For certain low energy β-emitters (for example ^{35}S, ^{14}C) this fraction may be rather small, unless a counter with a thinner window is used. Special thin-window counters are available for this purpose.

The avalanche associated with each pulse produces a dense region of space charge around the wire, with the negative charges (usually free electrons) moving towards the anode and being captured by it, and the positive ions moving outwards rather slowly (because of their lower mobility) towards the cathode. The existence of this 'sheath' implies that the arrival of a second β-particle before the charge has dispersed will not be able to form a further avalanche. This gives rise to 'dead time' which will typically be 150–200 μs. When dispersal of the charge is nearing completion, a newly-arrived β-particle may produce a pulse, though of reduced height, and because of the uncertainty associated with this, a preferred mode of operation is to 'quench' the counter momentarily by reducing the applied potential, during which time the system will be inactive for a definite period after each pulse. This time will be accurately constant from pulse to pulse, and is usually set to a value of about 400 μs. This dead-time sets a limit to the maximum counting rate at which the counter can be used. If the observed counting rate is N_{obs}, the system will be inoperative for a fraction of time $N_{obs}\tau$, where τ is the dead time (or paralysis time) imposed by the quenching circuit. The 'true' counting rate will then be given by

$$N_{true} = \frac{N_{obs}}{1 - N_{obs}\tau} \qquad (3.2)$$

This equation is used to correct the observed counts for counting losses, and we may speak of a 'percentage live time' given by

$$(1 - N_{obs}\tau) \times 100\%.$$

It is clear that the percentage live time declines significantly if the counting rate exceeds a few hundred counts per second, which accordingly sets an upper limit to the counting rate at which a Geiger counter may be used.

The filling gas is normally one of the rare gases, usually neon or argon. To this must be added a few percent of a 'quenching' gas, usually an organic vapour such as ethyl alcohol or ethyl formate. This is included in order to absorb any ultraviolet photons released during the avalanche and which would otherwise release further electrons from the electrodes, rendering the avalanche uncertain in magnitude and possibly precipitating a continuous discharge. The quenching gas has a second function, because the arrival of the positive ions at the cathode can, in principle, cause the release of further electrons, and this can cause the initiation of a second pulse. The presence of a quenching gas of relatively low ionization potential can prevent this, because the charge carried by the positive ions can be transferred to the quenching gas; the energy released at the point of impact with the cathode then causes the dissociation of the organic molecule rather than the release of an electron. In the halogen-quenched counter, a small percentage of chlorine or bromine performs the same function, and has the advantage that recombination of the dissociated halogen molecules (Cl_2, Br_2) appears to occur. The quenching gas is thus not used up, and the counters therefore have a longer life.

Geiger counters are normally used for the detection of β-radiation and, although they represent one of the earliest and simplest types of nuclear radiation detector, they remain widely used for all types of assay work in which activities of samples have to be measured and compared. The detection efficiency of a Geiger counter for γ-detection is low (1–2% only), but if one of the heavier noble gases (for example krypton) is used, the efficiency for x-rays becomes quite high, so that these detectors may be used effectively for the assay of electron capture isotopes.

Geiger counters made of thin glass, without a specially fabricated window, are useful in instruments designed for radiation monitoring. Other special types include one of glass construction, surrounded by a further glass envelope which may be filled with up to 7–8 ml of solution. These are known as liquid counters, and may be used for the higher energy β-emitters. They have the advantage that the sample for assay does not have to be prepared in solid form.

If the potential difference between the electrodes is somewhat reduced, the gas multiplication becomes less, and the avalanche no longer involves the whole wire. The amount of charge reaching the anode can now, in principle, be proportional to the number of initial ion-pairs formed, which in turn is proportional to the energy of the ionizing particle. This important property forms the basis of the **proportional counter** which is widely used for spectrometry of x-rays and low energy γ-rays, and is particularly useful when some discrimination is required between these radiations and higher energy γ-rays (Fig. 3.2).

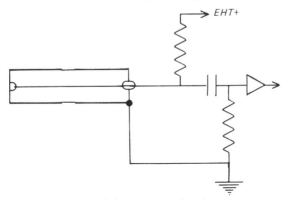

Fig. 3.2 The proportional counter

To achieve proportionality, the following design criteria must be met:

(a) The electric field must be accurately uniform around the wire. This requires a cylindrical geometry, and although the wire does not have to be coaxial to a high degree of accuracy, it must be accurately circular in cross-section, uniform in radius throughout its length, and free from any asperities or adherent dust particles.

(b) To ensure free mobility of the electrons, all traces of gases which have an affinity for electrons (oxygen, water vapour, oxides of nitrogen) must be rigorously excluded, by appropriate outgassing and by careful attention to gas purity.

(c) The EHT supply must be carefully stabilized (to 1 part in 10^4) because the gas multiplication factor varies very sensitively with field strength.

(d) The range of the ionizing particles released by the γ-ray interactions must be less than the linear dimension of the counter. Because no positive-ion sheath is formed around the wire, the recovery time of the counter is much faster than that of a Geiger counter. The counter can respond correctly to pulses separated by only a few microseconds, and so counting rates up to, and even beyond, 10^4 s^{-1} are practicable. The gas multiplication will not normally exceed about 10^3, and so the pulses are much smaller than those from a Geiger counter, being no more than a few millivolts in amplitude. These can be amplified without difficulty, but it is necessary to use a small preamplifier, connected to the counter using as short a lead as is practicable, in addition to the main amplifier, to avoid attaching too much electrical capacity to the counter itself.

The ability of a radiation detector to distinguish between photons (or particles) of closely similar energy is termed its **energy resolution**. For a proportional counter, this will depend on the statistical spread in the number of initial events, and also on the statistics of the multiplication process. We may examine the energy resolution of a proportional counter as follows:

Let

N = number of initial ion-pairs released by the ionizing particle
M = gas multiplication for 1 initial electron
$\bar{M}$ = mean value of M averaged over N initial electrons
P = *final* number of ion pairs per pulse

$\therefore$ $P = N\bar{M}$

For the relative variance of P, we may write

$$\left(\frac{\sigma_P}{P}\right)^2 = \left(\frac{\sigma_N}{N}\right)^2 + \left(\frac{\sigma_{\bar{M}}}{\bar{M}}\right)^2 \qquad (3.3)$$

If N is distributed according to a Poisson distribution,

$$\left(\frac{\sigma_N}{N}\right)^2 = \frac{1}{N}$$

In fact, the relative variance is less than this, and may be written as

$$\left(\frac{\sigma_N}{N}\right)^2 = \frac{F}{N},$$

where F is known as the Fano factor.

Furthermore

$$\left(\frac{\sigma_{\bar{M}}}{\bar{M}}\right)^2 = \frac{1}{N}\left(\frac{\sigma_M}{\bar{M}}\right)^2.$$

The quantity $\left(\frac{\sigma_M}{\bar{M}}\right)^2$ is difficult to evaluate theoretically. Because of the multiplicative nature of the process, we would not expect it to be small. It is found to be of the order of unity, and may be denoted by G.

$$\text{Hence} \quad \left(\frac{\sigma_P}{P}\right)^2 = \frac{F+G}{N} \tag{3.4}$$

F is dependent on a number of factors relating to the ionization processes, and is found to be in the region of 0.2. G has been determined experimentally by studying the multiplication of single electrons released by ultra-violet photons, and is found to be approximately 0.7.

Hence, to a close degree of approximation

$$\frac{\sigma_P}{P} \approx \frac{1}{\sqrt{N}} = \sqrt{\frac{W}{E_\gamma}} \tag{3.5}$$

W is approximately 26 eV for Argon, hence

$$\frac{\sigma_P}{P} \approx 0.16 \, E_\gamma^{-\frac{1}{2}} \quad (E \text{ in keV}) \tag{3.6}$$

Resolution is normally expressed as the full width of the peak (ΔP) at half maximum height ($FWHM$). This, for a gaussian distribution, is 2.35 σ.

Hence

$$\frac{\Delta P}{P} \approx 0.38 \, E_\gamma^{-\frac{1}{2}} \quad (E \text{ in keV}) \tag{3.6}$$

Results obtained from good counters conform generally to this form of expression. For example, for the K_α x-ray of manganese (5.9 keV), obtained from the electron capture isotope ^{55}Fe, a resolution ($FWHM$) of about 16% is typical. A proportional counter may be calibrated using a few x-ray sources of known photon energy, and is useful mainly in the energy range of 3–40 keV. Below 3 keV the energy resolution is not adequate for spectroscopy, although proportional counters fitted with especially thin windows, may be used (along with suitable crystals for spectroscopy by Bragg reflection), as radiation detectors for photon energies down to a few hundred eV.

Because of the relatively low mobility of the positive ions, the motion of charges in the counter does not cease until several hundred micro-seconds have elapsed since the arrival of the ionizing particle or γ-ray photon. The mobility of electrons is much greater; accordingly, only that part of the pulse caused by the electrons is used. In this connection the details of formation of the pulse are of some interest.

Referring to Fig. 3.3, we show some ion-pairs immediately after formation but before separation, and it is clear that a charge will begin to appear on the counter terminal as soon as charge separation begins. It is pertinent to ask what will be the effective charge q' at the terminal when the electrons have been collected, but before the positive ions have moved appreciably from the point of formation. This may be understood from the following argument:

Let the stored electrostatic energy in the system be denoted by E.

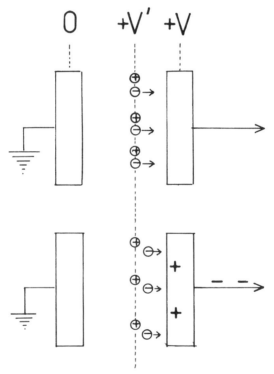

Fig. 3.3   Illustrating the movement of charge in an ion chamber or a proportional
counter immediately after the passage of a charged particle

Then, $E = \frac{1}{2}CV^2 = \frac{1}{2}\frac{Q^2}{C}$ (3.7)

Work done by the field in moving the charge $-q$ from potential $+V'$ to V

$$= +q\,(V - V')$$

$$\therefore \ \Delta E = -q\,(V - V')$$ (3.8)

This can also be written

$$\frac{1}{2}\frac{(Q - q')^2}{C} - \frac{1}{2}\frac{Q^2}{C}$$

$$= -\frac{Qq'}{C}$$ (3.9)

Hence, equating this with (3.8),

$$q' = \frac{q\,(V - V')}{V}$$ (3.10)

showing that the pulse produced by the motion of electrons is **proportional to the potential difference through which the charge falls.**

The gas multiplication all takes place very close to the wire. This means that the size of the pulse is only a small fraction of the maximum possible pulse height, but the rise time of the electron component is of the order of $1\,\mu S$ or less, enabling the system to be used as a fast counter. The fact that virtually all the electrons in an avalanche are produced close to the wire ensures that there will be no spread in pulse height on account of electrostatic considerations, and also that the pulse height will be independent of the position within the counter at which the initial ionizing event takes place.

The pulse shape appearing at the counter terminal is illustrated in Fig. 3.4. To reduce the duration of the slowly-varying part, the signal is passed through a differentiating time constant, the value of which should be just a little longer than the collection time of the electrons. It is also customary to follow this (through a suitable buffer amplifier) with an integrating time contact, which is chosen so as to be able to reduce electronic noise without seriously attenuating the signal.

One final point should be noted. When a photon is absorbed in the counter gas, it will normally ionize an atom in an inner shell, and this will result in the subsequent emission of an x-ray or an Auger electron. If an Auger electron is emitted, or if an emitted x-ray is absorbed elsewhere in the counter, the whole of the energy of the incident photon will contribute to the pulse. If however the x-ray escapes from the counter, the size of the pulse will be reduced by an amount which is proportional to the loss of energy. This will give rise to an 'escape peak' in the resulting pulse height distribution. This may be minimised by using a counter of large size. However, if a gas of moderately high atomic number is used (to facilitate high absorption of the incident radiation), the fluorescence yield will be high, and if additionally the counter is not sufficiently large, the escape peaks may be prominent and must then be taken into consideration when interpreting the pulse height distributions.

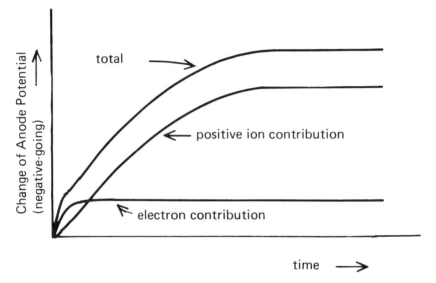

Fig. 3.4 The pulse shape at the output terminal of a proportional counter

3.3 THE SCINTILLATION COUNTER

The use of a radiation detector in solid form, especially for gamma radiation, is attractive because of the much higher detection efficiencies which can be achieved. The scintillation counter depends upon the luminescence which many materials exhibit when exposed to ionizing radiation. In an insulating solid, the electrons are normally confined to the valence band, but under the influence of ionizing radiation an electron may be raised into the conduction band. This electron may then fall into an electron trap (which possibility is discussed briefly in the reference to thermoluminescence in section 3.5) or may return immediately to the valence band. If, however, certain types of impurity atom are present, these may act as **luminescence centres**. Electrons crossing the band gap may combine with these centres, with the consequent emission of light. Optical photons generated in this way may then be detected by a photomultiplier in optical contact with the luminescent material. Scintillators which depend upon the presence of controlled amounts of added impurity are termed 'impurity-activated' materials. However, many organic materials, whether crystalline or liquid, exhibit luminescence in the pure form, and are therefore said to be 'intrinsic' in nature. We may thus distinguish two classes of scintillator in normal use: first the inorganic, impurity-activated crystals, the most common of which are sodium iodide (thallium activated) and caesium iodide (thallium or sodium activated); secondly, the organic scintillators, including certain aromatic crystals, notably anthracene, and more commonly, polymerised plastic materials which are available in a wide variety of machined shapes and sizes.

The excited ions (luminescence centres in an impurity-activated crystal) or molecules (in an organic scintillator) decay with finite life-time, known as the **luminescent decay time**. In organic materials, luminescent decay times tend to be short (5-20 nS) and such scintillators are widely used for fast counting of β-particles from solid samples or from radioactive solutions. In the inorganic crystals, which are used mainly for the measurement of γ-radiation, the decay times are somewhat longer. In sodium iodide, two components may be identified in the luminescent decay curve, with decay times of 0.23 μS and 1.5 μS. The pulse duration then is of the same order as for a gas proportional counter, and count rates up to $10^4 \, s^{-1}$ are readily achieved.

The number of optical photons released in the crystal is found to be proportional to the energy of the ionizing particle. The scintillation counter therefore can be used as a γ-ray spectrometer, if the incident γ-rays are absorbed with high efficiency, and if the whole of the energy of an incident photon is able to contribute to the production of optical photons by the luminescent process. This can be best achieved if the γ-ray is absorbed by the photoelectric process. To ensure this, it is necessary that at least some of the atoms comprising the crystal shall have a moderately high atomic number. Sodium iodide and caesium iodide fulfill this requirement.

A scintillation counter, then, consists essentially of a crystal in good optical contact with a photomultiplier, and is illustrated in Fig. 3.5. The crystal will normally be encapsulated, which is essential in the case of sodium iodide because it is highly deliquescent, and some light-scattering material will usually be incorporated around the crystal to ensure that the light is transmitted from the crystal to the photomultiplier with high efficiency. The photomultiplier consists of a photocathode, (at which a proportion of the optical photons are absorbed) followed by a series of dynodes, at each of which some electron multiplication takes place, by secondary electron emission. The signal reaching the anode following 10 or 12 such multiplication processes will exceed the initial number of electrons released at the cathode by a factor which will be typically of order 10^6. A pulse of 10-100 mV is produced, which is then amplified and passed to a single- or multi-channel analyser.

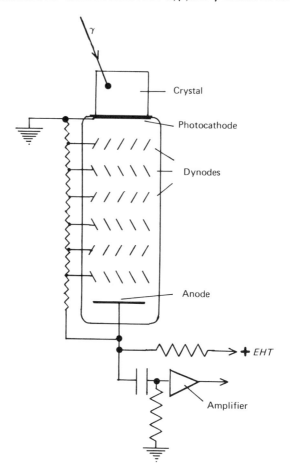

Fig 3.5 The scintillation counter, showing crystal, photomultiplier and anode connections

If photons are incident on the front surface of the crystal, the efficiency may be defined as the fraction of incident photons producing a pulse (of any size) in the photomultiplier anode circuit. Clearly the efficiency will depend upon crystal length, effective atomic number, and photon energy. It will also depend upon the degree of divergence of the beam (assuming that it originates from a point on the crystal axis), because of the occurrence of edge effects. For a parallel beam, the efficiency is shown in Fig. 3.6 for cylindrical crystals of three different lengths, (but all of the same radius), as a function of photon energy. Clearly the efficiency is high for much of the energy range of γ-rays encountered in practical radioactivity, but declines to somewhat low values for higher energies.

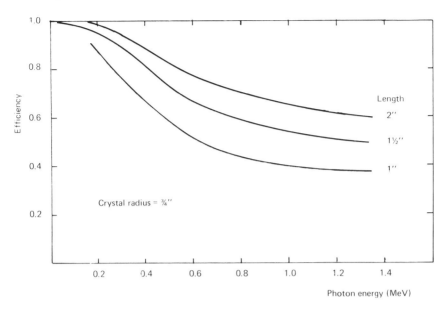

Fig. 3.6 Crystal efficiency (from data of Berger and Doggett (1956))

When a photon is absorbed, the interaction which deposits energy in the crystal may be either the photoelectric or the Compton effect. If the interaction is of the latter kind, only a portion of the energy of the photon will be deposited in the crystal, and the pulse produced will be of reduced height, with an upper limit which corresponds to the maximum amount of energy which may be transferred in a collision with a free electron. From (1.33) this may be seen to be

$$E_{max} = \frac{2E_\gamma^2}{2E_\gamma + mc^2} \tag{3.11}$$

The fraction of photoelectric interactions taking place will be given by

$$f = \frac{\sigma_{photo}}{\sigma_{photo} + \sigma_{compton} + \sigma_{pair\ production}} \tag{3.12}$$

and for a small crystal this fraction will represent the fraction of pulses which are of full height. For a crystal of practical size, however, there is a significant probability that the scattered photon will be absorbed in the crystal before reaching the crystal boundary; the full energy will thus be deposited in the crystal and the incident photon will contribute to the 'photoelectric peak' of the spectrum. The probability that a recorded event will appear in this peak is termed the **photofraction**. We may denote the product of the efficiency and the photofraction as the **photoelectric efficiency**.

The photofraction is illustrated, for crystals of 3 different sizes, in Fig. 3.7, from which it may be seen that a large crystal is advantageous in this respect.

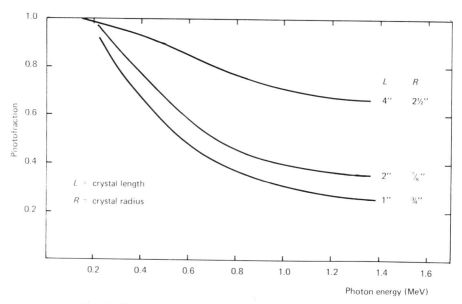

Fig. 3.7 Photofraction (from data of Berger and Doggett (1956))

It has been assumed that a photoelectric interaction ensures that the whole of the energy of the absorbed photon is deposited in the crystal. This is true in practice, because, although absorption in the K shell will produce a vacancy which has then to be filled by an outer electron, any Auger electrons emitted will be absorbed with certainty, and any x-rays emitted will be absorbed with high probability. X-ray 'escape peaks' are therefore not normally observed, although for relatively low energy γ-rays (absorbed near the surface of the crystal) the probability of x-ray escape is not quite negligible, and an escape peak may be visible.

If the incident photon has an energy which is substantially in excess of 1.02 MeV, a proportion of the interactions will take place by pair production. The subsequent annihilation of the positrons produce by these interactions will produce photons of 511 keV, the escape probability of which is substantial.

This effect gives rise to 'single' and 'double' escape peaks, corresponding to the escape of one or both annihilation photons. Fig. 3.8 illustrates the probability of escape of 0, 1, or 2 photons and shows that the predominant process may be any of these three alternatives, depending essentially on crystal size.

Fig. 3.9 illustrates the spectrum from the radioisotope ^{24}Na, from two crystals of different sizes. Photopeaks, single and double escape peaks, and the

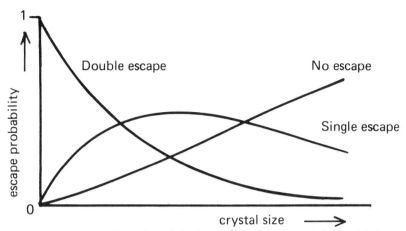

Fig. 3.8 Schematic illustration of the dependence of escape probability of 0, 1, or 2 annihilation photons on crystal size

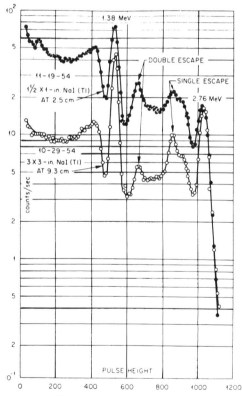

Fig. 3.9   Spectrum of ^{24}Na γ-radiation obtained with a scintillation counter, using sodium iodide crystals 1½″ × 1½″ (upper curve) and 3″ × 3″ (lower curve) (Neiler and Bell, 1965)

Compton continuum are all clearly seen, and the advantage of the larger crystal, in reducing the size of the escape peaks relative to the size of the main peaks, is clearly revealed.

The energy resolution of a scintillation counter depends upon the number, N, of electrons released at the photocathode, and on the statistical fluctuations in the electron multiplication process. A theoretical treatment can be developed in a manner somewhat similar to that used in the case of the proportional counter. Again it is found that

$$\frac{\sigma_P}{P} \approx \frac{1}{\sqrt{N}},$$

which is proportional to $E_\gamma^{-\frac{1}{2}}$. However, in a sodium iodide crystal, about 70 eV are expended, on average, for each optical photon produced, and the conversion efficiency at the photocathode is only in the region of 20%. The quantity analogous to W in (3.5) is therefore of the order of 350 eV, and so we may write

$$\frac{\sigma_P}{P} \approx 0.6\, E_\gamma^{-\frac{1}{2}} \quad (E_\gamma \text{ in keV})$$

and $$\frac{\Delta P}{P} \approx 1.4\, E_\gamma^{-\frac{1}{2}} \quad (E_\gamma \text{ in keV}); \tag{3.13}$$

the resolution is therefore inferior by a factor of about four, by comparison with a proportional counter. The two types of device are, however, normally used in different energy ranges – a scintillation counter is not normally used for spectrometry below about 50 keV, although if broad discrimination against electronic noise and high energy γ-radiation is all that is needed, it may be used with profit down to the region of 30 keV, for example for the detection and measurement of the radiation from ^{125}I (Te x-rays 28 keV; γ-transition 35 keV). At the energy of ^{137}Cs γ-radiation (662 keV), a good sodium iodide crystal can give a resolution of 7%.

Special types of scintillation counter have been developed for particular purposes. The 'well-type' crystal is cylindrical in form with a re-entrant cylindrical hole which can accommodate a small specimen tube capable of holding 7–10 ml of liquid. Suitably shielded, this forms a counter of great sensitivity, and activities down to a few nCi can be measured. For very low-energy β-emitters, notably tritium (E_β end-point = 17 keV), the scintillator may be an organic liquid, and the sample can be dissolved in it. This is practicable even if the sample is in aqueous solution, provided that the amount of added solution is small and that the 'quenching' of the scintillator (its reduction of light output) is measured if necessary by subsidiary experiments. As a final example, it may be pointed out that scintillators of large diameter (20–25 cm) and 1–2 cm in thickness are fabricated for use in scintillation cameras (see section 5.6).

No reference has yet been made to the use of scintillation counters for the measurement of α-particles. This may be achieved with the use of thin screens of zinc sulphide, which is very sensitive to α-particles. It must not be forgotten that this scintillator holds a position of high importance in the development of nuclear physics, having been used extensively in the period 1910–1930 for the quantitative study of α-radioactivity and the study of the 'historic' nuclear reactions under investigation at that time. Zinc sulphide has the property of being relatively opaque, but this is not a disadvantage for α-particle detection, where only thin screens are needed on account of the short range of α-particles, and the use of a detector of greater thickness than the particle range would result only in an increase of γ-ray background. Zinc sulphide scintillators, with photomultipliers, are used in α-particle detectors (for example for bench-top monitoring) and for specialised studies in connection with toxicity and hazards of α-emitting isotopes.

3.4 SOLID-STATE SEMICONDUCTOR DETECTORS

Semiconductor detectors have been in use in nuclear research for many years, and more recently they have found their way into applied nuclear and radiation physics laboratories, and into the field of medical physics.

In a semiconductor, electrons are normally to be found in the valence band, and no electrons (or very few) in the conduction band, which is separated from the valence band by the band gap. The width of this gap is 1.12 eV in silicon and 0.67 eV in germanium at room temperature, these two elements being the predominant materials used in semiconductor devices. These materials are normally poor conductors, but if an ionizing particle enters the material, electrons are raised into the conduction band and the system becomes momentarily conducting. If a field is applied across suitable electrodes the electron-hole pairs separate and move towards their respective electrodes, and a signal is formed. The rapid separation and collection of these charges is the situation to be aimed at in a good semiconductor radiation detector. The amount of electronic noise must be minimised, and this may be achieved by cooling the system to liquid nitrogen temperatures. Simple **conduction counters** may be made in this way, and have been used for the detection of α- and β-particles. Very high purity is required in such devices, because impurities can act as trapping centres, preventing the collection of charge. Diamond, cadmium telluride, and high resistivity silicon have been used for conduction counters.

We turn to a more important device, the **silicon surface-barrier detector**, which is in wide use for the detection of charged particles, and which can be operated at room temperature. This consists of an n-type silicon wafer, with a layer of p-type material at the surface, which may simply be the 'natural' surface covered with a thin gold film to provide ohmic contact. If this device is operated under reverse-bias conditions, all charge carriers will be swept out, and a 'depletion layer' of high resistivity is formed. An ionizing particle entering this layer will produce a signal, and if the particle is stopped completely in the depletion layer, the size of the signal is proportional to the particle energy. It is found that the mean energy necessary to produce an electron-hole pair is 3.5 eV in silicon. The number of charges collected is thus much greater than in the gas proportional counter, and so solid-state detectors have, in principle, much better energy resolution than the other detectors so far described; rapid development of the technology has led to a wide variety of solid-state detectors being available with energy resolutions consistent with theoretical expectations. α-particle spectrometry can be carried out with a surface-barrier detector, and heavier particles, including fission fragments, can be examined.

The thickness of these devices is normally limited to one or two millimetres, and so they are not practicable for use as γ-ray detectors. Furthermore, at γ-ray or x-ray energies sufficiently low to enable such a thin detector to be used, electronic noise generated within the detector would prevent the achievement of adequate energy resolution.

An important advance was secured when it was found possible to introduce impurity atoms into suitable semiconductor materials, by 'drifting' under the influence of heat and an applied electric field. In this type of detector, p-type silicon or germanium is provided with a surface layer of donor impurity atoms which can be drifted in to the material to form a material of very high resistivity. Lithium is commonly used for this purpose, and the lithium drifted silicon (Si(Li)) and germanium (Ge(Li)) detectors are widely used for x-ray and γ-ray spectrometry. In the Si(Li) detector, a resolution ($FWHM$) of 150 eV can be achieved in the 5–10 keV region (the 5.9 keV Mn K_α line emitted by ^{55}Fe is commonly used as a standard source for this work) and in germanium (for which $W = 2.94$ eV), resolutions of 1.5–2.0 keV are routinely possible, at photon energies of 0.5–1 MeV. Path lengths of several centimetres are practicable in Ge(Li) detectors, and so efficiencies comparable with the scintillation counter are possible, in this energy region.

The physical processes of γ-ray interaction are already familiar, and the spectrum of ^{24}Na illustrated in Fig. 3.10 may be interpreted in the same way as was described for the spectrum of the same radioisotope obtained with a scintillation counter (Fig. 3.9).

Lithium-drifted detectors must always be maintained at a low temperature, even when not in use, and therefore are mounted on a liquid-nitrogen Dewar vessel. This is a strict requirement — if the detector is allowed to warm up to room temperature, the lithium atoms can diffuse from their sites, and the functioning of the device is impaired. Cooling during use is in any case necessary in order to reduce noise levels (both in the detector and in the input circuit of the preamplifier) to acceptable values. A further difficulty is that they are subject to radiation damage, especially if used in a radiation environment which includes fast neutrons. These difficulties are overcome in part by the high-purity germanium detector, in which no 'drifting-in' of donor atoms is needed. These devices may be stored at room temperature, and are measurably more resistant to radiation damage than the lithium-drifted detectors. They must still, however, be cooled during use.

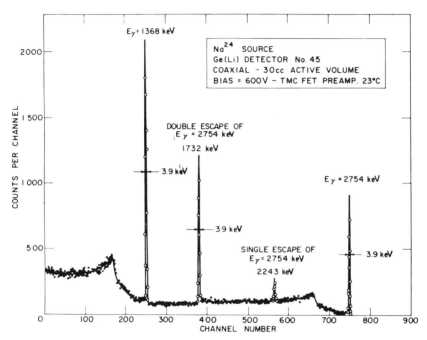

Fig. 3.10 Spectrum of ^{24}Na γ-radiation obtained using a Ge(Li) detector (Orphan and Rasmussen, 1967)

3.5 RADIATION DOSIMETRY

The purpose of radiation dosimetry is to establish the energy per unit mass absorbed from a field of ionizing radiation. The well-established unit for this purpose is the rad ('radiation absorbed dose') which is equal to 0.01 J per kilogram of any specified material. More recently, the S.I. unit (the gray) of 1 J $(kg)^{-1}$ has been introduced. One of the earliest observed effects of radiation from x-ray tubes and radioactive materials is its ability to ionize air in the vicinity of the source. The ionizing effect also lends itself to convenient instrumentation. It is not surprising therefore that radiation dosimetry consists largely of ionization dosimetry. Most of the material in this section will be concerned with ionization dosimetry, although we shall refer briefly to other methods. We begin by discussing the ionization dosimetry of x- and γ-radiation.

Consider a medium (for example carbon) immersed in a field of ionizing radiation. It will become suffused with electrons released by the gamma-ray interactions described in Chapter 1, and the energy distribution of these electrons will be determined by the physical details of these processes, as well as by the spectral distribution of the γ-radiation field. Let us now introduce a small cavity into the medium. If the cavity is sufficiently small, it is our contention that **the energy distribution and angular distribution of the electrons will be completely unchanged by this.** Let us now introduce a gas (which will often be air, though not necessarily so) into the cavity. The gas will become ionized, and in principle this ionization can be measured, for example by introducing electrodes and measuring the current flowing in an external circuit under the influence of a moderate applied potential. Let the energy absorbed per unit volume in the gas and in the solid by $_vE_g$ and $_vE_s$ respectively, and let the mean linear stopping powers for the electrons be $(dT/dx)_g$ and $(dT/dx)_s$ respectively.†

Then we may write

$$\frac{_vE_g}{_vE_s} = \frac{(dT/dx)_g}{(dT/dx)_s} \tag{3.14}$$

If the number of ion-pairs released per unit volume of gas be denoted by $_vJ$, and if W is the mean energy required to produce an ion-pair,

$$_vE_g = _vJW$$

Hence $$_vE_s = _vJW\frac{(dT/dx)_s}{(dT/dx)_g}$$

and if we now introduce the energy absorbed per unit mass $_mE_g$ and $_mE_s$, and the densities ρ_g and ρ_s, we get

$$\rho_s\cdot_mE_s = \rho_g\cdot_m JW\frac{(dT/dx)_s}{(dT/dx)_g}$$

or $$_mE_s = _m JW\frac{(dT/d(\rho x))_s}{(dT/d(\rho x))_g} \tag{3.15}$$

This is the formal statement of the **Bragg–Gray theorem.**

Clearly $_mJ$ can be equated to $\dfrac{Q}{eM}$, where Q is the total charge collected during the irradiation, e is the electronic charge, and M the total mass of gas in the cavity. We assume complete collection of the ion-pairs produced.

† In this section we use T to denote electron kinetic energy, reserving E for the (macroscopic) energy absorbed in a solid medium or a gas.

We have thus obtained a relationship between absorbed dose in a solid, and the ionization current in a gas. The only quantities required are the specific energy losses $dT/d(\rho x)$ for gas and solid, and W.

Let us consider the fundamental assumptions we have made in the course of this argument.

1. The electron spectrum is not affected by the presence of the cavity, that is, the energy loss sustained by any electron crossing the cavity is small, and the dimensions of the cavity are small compared with the range of the electrons in the gas.

2. Photon interactions generating electrons **in the gas** are negligible.

3. The spatial photon flux around the cavity is uniform.

In addition we have made the practical assumptions that (a) sufficient is known about the electron energy spectrum to enable the ratio of mean stopping powers to be calculated with adequate accuracy and (b) the quantity W is independent of electron energy, or at least that its value is known for the distribution of electron energies relevant to the experimental situation.

However, within the limits of these assumptions, (3.15) is rigorously correct for any combination of solid and gas.

We may ask what restrictions the photon energy E_γ places on the result. Clearly the criterion of small cavity size is easier to satisfy at higher values of E_γ, because the range of the secondary electrons will then be greater. But it is also necessary for electronic equilibrium to be established at the cavity, which, broadly speaking, means that there must be a thickness of material on all sides of the cavity at least equal to the range of the fastest electrons released by the incident photons. This requirement may cause some attenuation of the flux. If we now think of the solid as forming the walls of a cavity ionization chamber, it is clear that the current would vary with wall thickness somewhat as illustrated in Fig. 3.11 and that measurements with various wall thicknesses, combined with extrapolation to zero thickness, must be carried out, in order to obtain a valid result.

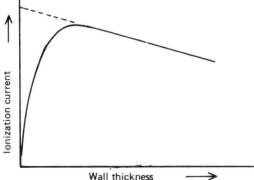

Fig. 3.11 Current in an ionization chamber as a function of wall thickness

The Bragg–Gray equation therefore solves the general problem of determining the absorbed dose in any material which can be fabricated into the walls of an ionization chamber. It may therefore be used to determine dose in any material (for example water, biological tissues, chemical systems, structural materials being studied for radiation damage, etc.) providing that the ratio of the **mass energy-absorption coefficients** for the chamber walls and the material under investigation is known.

In practice it is convenient to design the chamber so that its walls are not too different in effective atomic number from the material in which the absorbed dose is to be determined. For example, various conducting plastics have been devised which are approximately equivalent to biological tissue, so that absorption corrections can be applied with good accuracy, and so that, once calculated, they may be applicable over a wide range of incident photon energies.

Small ionization chambers of the type illustrated in Fig. 3.12 are in wide use for dosimetric work, in connection with diagnostic and therapeutic x-ray measurements. Ionization dosimetry requires the measurement of very small currents, down to 10^{-14} A, and the development and gradual improvement of electrometers (essentially D.C. amplifiers with an input resistance of the order of 10^{12} ohms) for this purpose has been of crucial importance in the establishment of good standards of dosimetry.

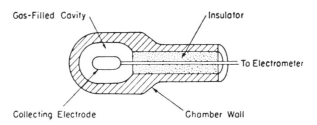

Fig. 3.12 Cavity ionization chamber (Attix *et al.*, 1966–9)

An important property of a beam of x- or γ-radiation is its **ionizing power in air**. This provides some information about the beam's ability to transfer energy to matter placed in its path and is relevant in the context of medical and biological work, because the effective atomic number of biological tissue does not differ substantially from that of air. The traditional unit of ionization *in air* is the **roentgen**. (It is not defined for any other gas.) Its definition was originally based on the old electrostatic unit (e.s.u.) of electric charge, and it was defined as the quantity of x- or γ-radiation which causes the liberation of 1 e.s.u. of charge of either sign per 0.001293 g of dry air. In terms of modern units, this corresponds to 2.58×10^{-4} C $(kg)^{-1}$ of charge liberated in air, which may, accordingly, be taken as the modern definition of the roentgen. We may readily calculate that an 'exposure' of 1 roentgen corresponds to an absorbed radiation dose of 0.869 rad $(0.869 \times 10^{-2} \text{ J (kg)}^{-1})$ in air. If the ratio of the mass energy-absorption coefficients of tissue to air be used as a multiplier, the absorbed dose in tissue may be calculated to be approximately 0.95 rad. Because the absorption in both these media is due almost entirely to the Compton effect, the ratio of absorbed doses will be very close to the ratio of the number of electrons per unit mass in the two media, which in turn is equal to the ratio of Z/A. It is thus almost independent of γ-ray energy in the range 0.1–3 MeV. Conversion factors relating the roentgen to the absorbed dose in several media are given in Table 3.2. In the case of soft tissue, the constancy of these factors over a wide range of energy will be noted, but, in contrast we see that in the case of bone, the relatively high Z causes large departures from this generalisation. In particular, the absorbed dose in bone may greatly exceed the value for organic material placed in the same beam. A consequence of this is that the dose imparted to small regions of soft tissue *within the bony structure* will also be substantially in excess of the value for extended regions of the same tissue. The small regions of tissue may in fact be treated as Bragg–Gray cavities surrounded by mineral bone. The dosimetry of bone and the soft tissue enclosed in it (the marrow) is important in connection with the determination of dose to the erythropoietic (red-cell forming) tissues in certain radiotherapeutic procedures. It has been extensively discussed by Spiers (1968).

Chambers designed on the Bragg–Gray principle, and with air-equivalent walls, are widely used to measure exposure in roentgens, or in C $(\text{kg})^{-1}$, but it is clear that to designate a beam in terms of 'rads in air' is just as satisfactory.

Table 3.2

Conversion factors from exposure to absorbed dose (rads/roentgen).
(Holm and Berry, 1970)

Photon energy (MeV)	Water	Muscle	Compact bone
0.01	0.912	0.925	3.55
0.02	0.879	0.917	4.23
0.04	0.879	0.920	4.14
0.06	0.905	0.929	2.91
0.08	0.932	0.940	1.91
0.1	0.949	0.949	1.46
0.5	0.965	0.957	0.925
1	0.965	0.957	0.919
2	0.965	0.955	0.921
3	0.962	0.955	0.929

The designation in terms of ionization per unit mass is therefore declining. No name has yet been assigned to the S.I. Unit 1 C $(kg)^{-1}$, and it is expected that this, and also the roentgen, will fall into disuse.

In order to measure absorbed dose at higher energies (for example the x-ray output from linear accelerators and betatrons) electronic equilibrium becomes progressively more difficult to achieve. In these circumstances it is sometimes found desirable to design the chamber with a *thin* wall, and to surround it completely with material as closely equivalent to the medium as is possible. In this way, the dose at points at various depths within the medium can be measured, and this, of course, is what is usually required in a practical situation.

In order to determine the roentgen by an absolute method, the 'free-air' chamber is used. The illustration in Fig. 3.13 will make clear the principle on which this is based. The ionization current is collected from an irradiated region of air of accurately defined volume. It is essential that electronic equilibrium be achieved so that electrons generated within the volume and leaving the system are balanced statistically by those entering the system from outside. Bearing in mind that the range of a 250 keV electron in air is approximately 50 cm, it will be clear that a free-air chamber installation requires to be of considerable size; these are, in fact, to be found only in the national standardising laboratories.

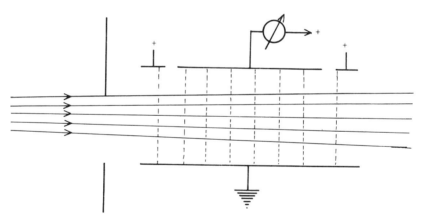

Fig. 3.13 The free air chamber

Referring back to (3.15), it will be appreciated that the relationship takes on a particularly simple form if the electronic mass stopping-powers of walls and gas are equal. Such a chamber is termed a **homogeneous** chamber, and it will be apparent that the Bragg–Gray conditions are now relaxed, in that the cavity no longer needs to be of small size. In circumstances where small size in the Bragg–Gray sense is inconvenient to achieve, homogeneous chambers have considerable advantages.

A few practical points may be noted:

(a) The potential difference applied to an ionization chamber should be sufficient to bring about complete separation of ion-pairs ('saturation') but not so large as to cause further ionization by collision. Furthermore, all sharp points and thin wires must be avoided in the interior of an ionization chamber, to prevent the occurence of localized regions of high field strength.

(b) Electronic equilibrium must be attained in the cavity by designing the walls to be sufficiently thick, or by varying the wall thickness and extrapolating, as already described.

(c) The possibility of recombination of ions has to be considered. We distinguish between **initial** and **general** recombination. Initial recombination is the recombination of ions which are formed initially in the same cluster or column. It is independent of dose rate, but increases with increasing LET of the secondary particles. It is negligible for electrons, in fields of the order of 100 V (cm)^{-1}. General recombination is the recombination of ions formed by different events. It is dependent on dose-rate, and may be significant at high dose-rates.

Turning briefly to the dosimetry of electron beams, this has become important in connection with the use of such beams for electron therapy, in which the particular depth-dose distribution associated with electrons can be of value in radiotherapy. It is also of importance in some areas of solid-state physics, for example research in thermoluminescence, and is significant in certain practical technologies, such as the bacterial sterilization of surgical instruments following manufacture and packaging.

Again we are interested in the absorbed dose, and for this purpose a cavity chamber may again be used. It would normally have a thin wall and be immersed in a medium equivalent to that in which the dose is to be determined. The electron spectrum will not be modified appreciably if the cavity is small. The chamber may be calibrated by converting it to a thick-walled chamber, and using a gamma-radiation field for a calibration measurement. Calibration is carried out in terms of absorbed dose. The roentgen (and indeed the whole concept of 'exposure' as a physical quantity) is confined to x- and γ-radiation, and is not defined for any other type of radiation.

Although ionization dosimetry is the most widely-used method for determination of absorbed dose, other methods exist, and it would be misleading to make no reference at all to these. However, they must be regarded as being marginal to the field implied by the title of this book, and so our discussion will be brief, and for a full account the reader is referred to the literature listed in the bibliography.

Dosimetry using **photographic film** has been carried out since the early days of x-rays, and, with good control of processing, allied to good densitometric measurement of the developed films, it has a useful and important role in radiation physics. It is an integrating method, measuring dose received over a long period of time, and has been used extensively in connection with radiation protection, where portability of film, and its ability to store information over a long period, both before and after development, have obvious advantages. Film can be used for both β- and γ-radiation, and the photographic technique can be extended to other radiations. One particular application is in mixed field dosimetry, particularly with mixed fields of fast neutrons and γ-radiation. In Chapter 6 we discuss briefly methods of neutron dosimetry, and it is shown that ionization chambers can be designed to give good absolute information on fast neutron dose. However, correction for the associated γ-ray dose is required, and although this can be achieved by taking simultaneous measurements using a second, neutron-insensitive ionization chamber, it is often preferable to use photographic film for this purpose.

It should be noted that film cannot give absolute information regarding dose, but must be calibrated with reference to standard radioactive sources, or ionization chambers.

The transfer of energy from a field of radiation to matter necessarily results in a small temperature rise, and this is the basis of **calorimetric** methods of dosimetry. A simple calculation will show that an absorbed dose of, say, 1000 rads, (sufficient to be lethal if given as a whole-body dose to mammals or the human subject), will produce a temperature rise of only a few millidegrees. The development of calorimetric dosimetry, at least for γ-radiation has depended upon the development of methods of accurately measuring very small temperature rises. The great importance lies in the fact that calorimetric dosimetry is an absolute method, requiring only that the specific heat and temperature rise of the medium be known. It thus provides an important check on ionization dosimetry.

To carry out an experiment in calorimetric dosimetry it is necessary to set up a sample (for example water or graphite) in a thermostatically-controlled enclosure, thermally insulated from its surroundings. Small temperature drifts cannot be wholly avoided, and the measurement of a temperature rise of the order of 10^{-2}-10^{-1} K to an accuracy of 1% require that the temperature drift of the system be followed before and after the irradiation, in order to carry out an extrapolation procedure along the lines indicated schematically in Fig. 3.14. In the **adiabatic** calorimeter the calorimeter itself may be surrounded by a water jacket maintained at the same temperature as the calorimeter by a heating system controlled by the *difference* in temperature between the calorimeter and the jacket. The changes in temperature can be measured by using thermistors (which have a high (negative) temperature coefficient of resistivity) in a bridge circuit. In this way, temperature changes can be measured to an accuracy which is in the region of 10^{-4} K. Various precautions have to be taken to ensure a reliable and accurate result, including the possibility of radiochemical reactions which modify — usually by reducing slightly — the observed temperature changes. This 'radiochemical defect' can be reduced by pre-irradiation of the system. Calorimetric dosimetry has been reviewed by Holm and Berry (1970), and a series of measurements has been reported by Bewley (1963) in whose paper the technical aspects of calorimetric dosimetry are closely examined.

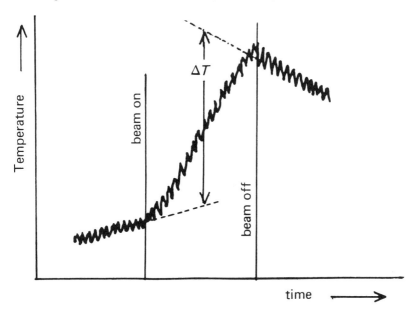

Fig. 3.14 Schematic illustration of temperature as a function of time in a calorimetric dosimeter

A further dosimetric technique, which is growing rapidly in importance, uses the phenomenon of **thermoluminescence**. We have seen in section 3.3 that the presence of impurities greatly affects the luminescent behaviour of solids. In thermoluminescent materials some of the electrons raised to the conduction band during irradiation fall into localised electron 'traps', which may be defects or vacancies in the crystal lattice. These electrons may remain trapped for long periods, but can be released by heating. During the heating a proportion of these electrons will recombine with luminescence centres, emitting light in the process. In many circumstances the total amount of light is proportional to the radiation dose, and the technique is becoming extensively used for field mapping in radio-therapy, and for radiation monitoring. Special materials (CaF_2, $CaSO_4$, LiF) doped with suitable impurities have been developed and can be used as small 'sachets' containing a few milligrams of powder, or as discs of the thermo-luminescent material embedded in PTFE (Teflon). Doses down to 20 mrad may be measured by thermoluminescent dosimetry, in connection with radiation protection. For mixed field dosimetry, thermoluminescent discs can be fabricated from LiF made from the separated isotopes ^{6}Li and ^{7}Li. Lithium fluoride made from ^{6}Li is very sensitive to neutrons, because of the high cross-section

(945 barns for thermal neutrons) of the $^6Li(n,\alpha)^3H$ reaction, whereas ^7LiF is relatively insensitive to neutrons. Both are, of course, equally sensitive to γ-radiation. Thermoluminescence is an interesting blend of solid-state physics and radiation physics, and its use in medical and biological applications will steadily increase.

The remaining field to be referred to here is that of **chemical dosimetry**. The rate at which chemical reactions take place can be modified by ionizing radiation, and in certain situations, particularly reactions involving oxidation or reduction, the process will occur to an extent proportional to the radiation dose received, and will occur only very slowly, or not at all, if ionizing radiation is absent. The 'Fricke' dosimeter consists of ferrous sulphate in sulphuric acid solution. Irradiation of samples of solution in small glass or plastic containers causes a series of chemical changes which, in essence, amount to the oxidation process $Fe^{2+} \rightarrow Fe^{3+}$. The Fe^{3+} can be determined by titration or by optical absorption spectroscopy, and the method is very suitable for determining radiation doses in the range 4×10^3–4×10^4 rads.

A quantitative reaction of this type is characterised by its 'G' value, which is the number of ions formed (or reacting) per 100 eV of absorbed energy. For the $Fe^{2+} \rightarrow Fe^{3+}$ reaction in the presence of oxygen the G value is 15.5. It is independent of γ-ray energy over a wide range (falling somewhat at lower photon energies – it becomes 13.8 for 10 keV x-rays) and is independent of dose rate between 0.1 and 4000 rad sec^{-1}. It is thus of great value as a dosimeter, especially for use in investigations in the field of radiation chemistry.

For the measurement of higher doses, the ceric sulphate dosimeter may be used. This is a reduction process, essentially $Ce^{4+} \rightarrow Ce^{3+}$ (although is carried out in aerated solution) and is useful in the range 10^4–10^8 rads. The G value is 2.44, and a linear response is reported between 10^5 and 10^7 rads. A further example is the decomposition of oxalic acid

$$COOH\text{-}COOH \rightarrow 2CO_2 + H_2$$

which is used in applied radiation work at very high radiation levels (10^6–10^8 rad). It may be used in the interior of a nuclear reactor, and has the advantage of not being subject to neutron activation.

In addition to the three quantitative chemical systems just described, many other quasi-chemical systems, based on colour changes or darkening, are known and are used. For details we refer the reader to the specialist literature on radiation dosimetry (see Bibliography).

In this section we have set out the principles of radiation dosimetry for external sources of γ-radiation and electrons. Other aspects of dosimetry are introduced elsewhere in this book – dosimetry in relation to the activity of radioactive sources is discussed in section 4.8; the internal dosimetry of radio-isotopes distributed in biological tissue is introduced in section 5.9; and the

dosimetry of fast neutrons is treated in section 6.4. The basic principles set out
in this section are, however, relevant to these other topics, and are necessary for
a full understanding of all aspects of radiation dosimetry.

FURTHER READING

Holm, N. W. and Berry, R. J. (Eds.) (1970) *Manual on Radiation Dosimetry*
Dekker
Price, W. J. (1964) *Nuclear Radiation Detection* McGraw-Hill
Siegbahn, K. (Ed.) (1965) α-, β-, and γ-ray Spectroscopy N. Holland Publishing
Co.

REFERENCES

Attix, F. H., Roesch, W. C. and Tochilin, E. (1966-9). See Further Reading for
Chapter 4
Berger, M. J. and Doggett, J. (1956) *J. Res. Nat. Bur. Stand.,* **56**, 355
Bewley, D. K. (1963) *Brit. J. Radiol,* **36**, 865
Neiler, J. H. and Bell, P. R. (1965) in Siegbahn, K. (Ed.), above
Orphan, W. J. and Rasmussen, N. C. (1967) *Nucl. Instr. Meth.* **48**, 282
Spiers, F. W. (1968) *Radioisotopes in the Human Body* Academic Press

The radiation from nuclear decay

4.1 α-DECAY

The α-particle is a strongly-bound body, with a total binding energy of 28 MeV which is about 7 MeV per nucleon. Referring to Fig. 2.2, we see that above an atomic mass of about 60, the binding energy per nucleon declines slowly with increasing A. This suggests that for A greater than some critical value, all nuclei will, in principle, be unstable against α-emission, because the relatively small amount of energy needed to allow the α-particle to form can readily be supplied by the increased binding energy of the remaining nucleons which form the daughter nucleus. Detailed analysis shows that in fact all nuclei with $A \gtrsim 150$ are α-unstable. However, the energy which the outgoing α-particle needs in order to penetrate the Coulomb barrier with measurable probability is such that α-emission is only rarely observable for atomic masses less than $A \sim 200$. Above this limit, many natural radioelements are to be found, and we recognise 3 natrually-occurring radioactive series, designated as the Thorium $(4n)$, Uranium-radium $(4n+2)$ and Uranium-actinium $(4n+3)$ series, to which the Neptunium $(4n+1)$ series has more recently been added, n being an integer. The parent element (^{237}Np) of the last series has a half-life of 2.2×10^6 years, which is much less than the age of the Universe. ^{237}Np is therefore extinct. It can, however, be produced artificially, and so the $(4n+1)$ series is now well-documented.

The emission of an α-particle may lead to a daughter nuclide which is β-unstable (on account of its neutron-to-proton ratio being somewhat increased by the loss of the α-particle) and therefore a series of α-decay processes interspersed with β-emission becomes the established pattern. For example, the transformation of $^{238}_{92}$U into its stable end-product $^{206}_{82}$Pb involves the emission of 8 successive α-particles and 6 β-particles.

It was early recognised that there is a strong inverse relationship between α-particle energy and life-time. Geiger and Nuttall established experimentally a power law of the form

$$\ln t_{1/2} = \text{const.} + \ln R \tag{4.1}$$

where $t_{1/2}$ and R are the half-life of the α-emitter and the range of the α-particle respectively. However, more recent work, and also the theoretical treatment outlined below, leads to a somewhat different relationship, and the Geiger–Nuttall law must be regarded as an empirical law, valid only over a somewhat limited range of the particle energies.

To understand the process of α-decay, it is necessary to consider the potential experienced by the α-particle (energy E_α) both inside and outside the nucleus (Fig. 4.1), interpreting the behaviour of the α-particle in terms of quantum mechanics. The α-particle may enter regions of the potential such that $V > E$, which classically are not accessible to it, and so may emerge from the nucleus with finite probability. This 'tunnelling effect' is such that the probability decreases with increasing barrier height and decreasing particle energy. The solution of the wave equation leads to a 'barrier penetration factor' of the form $e^{-2\epsilon}$, where ϵ can be expressed approximately as

$$\epsilon = \frac{\pi z Z e^2}{\hbar v} \tag{4.2}$$

where Z, e, and $\hbar$ have their usual meanings, $z\ (= 2)$ is the atomic number of the α-particle and v is the velocity of the α-particle after it has left the vicinity

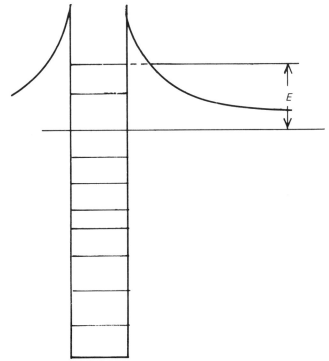

Fig. 4.1 Nuclear potential well, as seen by an α-particle of energy E

of the nucleus (that is $E_\alpha = \frac{1}{2} m_\alpha v^2$). If the decay is expressed in the form of the decay constant, λ, this would be expected to be proportional to the barrier penetration factor, enabling us to write

$$\lambda = \text{const.} \times e^{-2\epsilon} \qquad (4.3)$$

or $\qquad \ln \lambda = a - 2\epsilon = a - bE_\alpha^{-\frac{1}{2}}. \qquad (4.4)$

This law of variation of the decay constant with α-particle energy has been verified over a wide range of life-times, and illustrates the applicability of the quantum-mechanical tunnelling process to this problem, in which the life-times which can be observed experimentally range from ThC$'$ (^{212}Po) with a half-life of 3×10^{-7} s to such long-lived nuclides as ^{238}U ($t_{\frac{1}{2}} = 4.5 \times 10^9$ y), a factor of 10^{23}. The α-decay energies vary by only a factor of 3 or so, and for expected decay energies of less than about 3 MeV, the decay constants are usually unobservably small.

It should be added that many α-emitters can be made artificially which do not occur in any of the radioactive series referred to above.

α-emitters are not frequently encountered in biological applications, but are nevertheless of potentially great interest in radiobiological research, where the differing Relative Biological Efficiency ($q.v.$) of different radiations has a fundamental bearing on the biological effects of radiation at the cellular level. The high specific energy-loss of α-particles (see sections 1.2 and 1.3) is of significance here; for example, α-emitting isotopes of astatine ($Z = 85$) are of interest because of the chemical reactivity of astatine and because it is a chemical homologue of iodine.

The most familiar α-emitter is radium–226, which generates a series of α-, β-, and γ-emitting daughter products. Radium in equilibrium with its decay products is used in radiotherapy as a γ-emitter in the form of sealed platinum tubes or 'needles' (to prevent the external emission of α- or β-radiation and to trap gaseous products), and its specific γ-emission (section 4.8) has been carefully determined. It is important as a standard of radioactivity, because it can be prepared in a chemically and isotopically pure form; furthermore, its long half-life (1622 y) implies that standards can be accurately prepared on the basis of accurate weighing. Its use in radiotherapy is, however, declining; radium tubes and radium needles have to be checked periodically for leakage, and the use of α-emitters is now considered to present an unnecessary hazard, particularly as one of the members of the decay chain is a gas. Alternative γ-emitters, for example ^{192}Ir, are available which are free from these hazards.

4.2 β-DECAY

β-decay is by far the commonest form of a radioactive decay, and is a consequence of the 'weak interaction' between light particles (or 'leptons', which include electrons, positrons, neutrinos, and μ-mesons) and other matter. β-decay in radioactivity can take three forms – the emission of β^- or β^+ particles, or the absorption, by the nucleus, of an atomic electron, this process being known as orbital electron capture. To establish the circumstances in which β-decay is energetically possible we may proceed as follows:

Let M_Z be the mass of a **neutral atom** of element Z, and let E_β and $E_{\bar{\nu}}$ be the energies of the β-particle and antineutrino emitted in β^- decay.

Element Z decays to element $Z + 1$, with the emission of a β-particle and an antineutrino. Because energy is conserved in the β-decay, we may write

$$M_Z c^2 = M_{(Z+1)} c^2 + E_{\beta-} + E_{\bar{\nu}} \qquad (4.5)$$

The rest mass of the emitted β-particle does not appear on the right hand side of (4.5) because the electron released in the process, together with the Z electrons already present in the system, make up the $Z + 1$ electrons required for a neutral atom of element $Z + 1$.

If the difference between **atomic** mass-energies is denoted by Q, we see that for this process to be energetically possible,

$$Q > 0. \qquad (4.6)$$

For β^+ emission we may write

$$\text{element } Z \;\to\; \text{element } (Z - 1) + \beta^+ + \nu.$$

Hence $M_Z c^2 = M_{(Z-1)} c^2 + m_- c^2 + m_+ c^2 + E_\beta^+ + E_\nu$. For this process to occur

$$Q > 2mc^2, \qquad (4.7)$$

if we put $m_- = m_+$.

For electron capture,

$$\text{element } Z \;\to\; \text{element } (Z - 1) + \nu + E_{K, L...}$$

where $E_{K, L...}$ represents the excitation energy of the daughter $(Z - 1)$ atom, singly-ionized in its K, L... shell following electron capture. Noting that there are $(Z - 1)$ electrons associated with this atom, we may write:

$$M_Z c^2 = M_{(Z-1)} c^2 + E_\nu + E_{K, L...} \qquad (4.8)$$

and, for decay by this process to occur,

$$Q > E_{K, L...}. \qquad (4.9)$$

It will be apparent from these simple considerations that electron capture will always, in principle, occur as an alternative to positron emission. The two processes very often occur in the same radioisotope, with a branching ratio (that is relative probability) determined by Q and Z. Furthermore, if $E_K > Q > E_L$, capture from the L shell will be possible even though K capture is not. This would be revealed by the nature of the x-ray spectrum associated with the reversion of the excited atom to its ground state. The K spectrum would in fact be absent from the emitted x-rays.

Finally it should be added that, although the radioactive decay process is determined by the position of the nuclides on the curves of the type illustrated in Fig. 2.4, it is clear that, in the case of odd-odd nuclides, both alternatives (β^- and β^+ emission) may be energetically possible. Several examples of this are known, in which both alternatives occur with measurable probability (for example ^{64}Cu, ^{126}I).

The β-radiation forms a continuous spectrum, and the shape of the spectrum is determined by the probability that each particle shall be emitted into a certain interval of momentum. The Fermi statistical theory of β-decay examines this situation quantitatively, establishing that the probability, dn, of a β-particle of momentum p and a neutrino of momentum q being emitted simultaneously into momentum intervals dp and dq (respectively) is given by

$$dn = S_1 \frac{4\pi p^2}{h^3} dp \frac{4\pi q^2}{h^3} dq \qquad (4.10)$$

where S_1 is a weighting factor, which is equal to 4 for positron or electron emission to allow for the fact that each emitted particle has two possible directions of spin. That is, two particles of each kind can be emitted into a volume h^3 of momentum space.

Noting that $q = \dfrac{E_\nu}{c} = \dfrac{E_0 - E_\beta}{c}$,   and that

dq may be written as $\left(\dfrac{\partial q}{\partial E_0}\right)_{E_\beta} dE_0$ or as $\dfrac{dE_0}{c}$, $\qquad (4.11)$

we can write

$$dn = S_1 \frac{4\pi p^2 dp}{h^3} \cdot \frac{4\pi (E_0 - E_\beta)^2}{h^3 c^2} \cdot \frac{dE_0}{c}. \qquad (4.12)$$

It is shown in texts on quantum mechanics that the probability per unit time of decay into a particular momentum interval dp is given by

$$P(p)dp = \frac{dn}{dE_0} \times \frac{2\pi}{\hbar} \times |M|^2 \times g^2 . dp \qquad (4.13)$$

where $\dfrac{\mathrm{d}n}{\mathrm{d}E_0}$ is the density of states, $|M|^2$ is a matrix element expressing the degree of overlap between the nuclear wave functions of the initial and final states, and g^2 expresses the strength of the fundamental interaction involved in the process, which in the present problem is the 'weak' interaction characteristic of β-decay. We may therefore write this probability per unit time as

$$P(p)\mathrm{d}p \;=\; \frac{2\pi}{\hbar}|M|^2 g^2 S_1 \,\frac{16\pi^2 p^2 (E_0 - E_\beta)^2}{h^6 c^3}\,\mathrm{d}p. \tag{4.14}$$

This is often written in terms of p/mc and $(E - E_\beta)/mc^2$, and in this form the expression on the RHS of this equation becomes

$$\frac{2\pi}{\hbar}|M|^2 g^2 S_1 \,\frac{16\pi^2 m^5 c^4}{h^6}\left[\left(\frac{p}{mc}\right)^2 \cdot \left(\frac{E_0 - E_\beta}{mc^2}\right)^2 \cdot \mathrm{d}\left(\frac{p}{mc}\right)\right] \tag{4.15}$$

The quantity in square brackets, when modified by Coulomb effects of attraction or repulsion as the β^- or β^+ particle leaves the nucleus, and when integrated over all β-particle energies E_β from 0 to E_0, is often written as the function $f(E_0, Z)$, enabling us to write

$$P \;=\; g^2 |M|^2 S_1 \,\frac{m^5 c^4}{\hbar^7 2\pi^3}\, f(E_0, Z) \tag{4.16}$$

P may be identified as the decay constant of the transition, which is equal to $\ln 2/t_{1/2}$, where $t_{1/2}$ is the half-life.

We see that the quantity $ft_{1/2}$ is proportioned to $|M|^{-2}$. This quantity ranges over many orders of magnitude, and the higher values correspond to higher degrees of 'forbiddenness' of decay and hence to smaller values of the matrix element $|M|^2$. These smaller values are associated with larger changes, ΔI, of nuclear moment, I, in the β^- decay. The recorded half-lives of nuclides decaying by β-emission range from 10^{-2} s to 10^7 y. Doubtless nuclides exist with half-lives outside this range, but are unrecorded in the literature simply because of the practical problems involved in observing their decay.

We therefore expect the β^- decay of a given nuclide to occur with a characteristic half-life, and with a continuous spectrum of β-particles the shape of which depends on E, Z, and ΔI. The modification of spectral shape caused by Coulomb effects is illustrated in Fig. 4.2.

In the above discussion it has been supposed that the decay occurs to the ground state of the product (daughter) nucleus. If one or more excited states are populated, the decay constant, λ_d,† of the process is the sum of the individual

---

† Denoted in this and the following section as λ_d, to avoid confusion with wavelength λ.

constants λ_{d_1}, λ_{d_2}, etc., obtained from (4.16) for each group of β-particles. The subsequent decay of the excited states takes place with the emission of γ-radiation, which we now proceed to discuss.

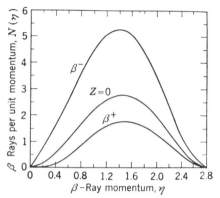

Fig. 4.2   Shape of 'allowed' beta-spectrum showing the effect of the coulomb forces on negatively and positively charged β-particles (β^- and β^+) (Evans, 1955)

4.3 γ-RADIATION

The emission of γ-radiation is an electromagnetic process determined by the distribution of charges and currents within the nucleus. Changes in these distributions are responsible for the emission of the electromagnetic radiation. The nucleus behaves like an oscillator of frequency $\nu = (E_i - E_f)/h$, and with a decay constant λ_d given by Γ/h, where Γ is the width of the state from which the transition proceeds. The decay constant is the probability per unit time of decay taking place, and is determined by the multipolarity and the character (electric or magnetic) of the transition. The behaviour of an oscillating electric multipole (dipole, quadrupole) is treated in texts on electromagnetic theory (for example Becker, 1964), and the power radiated can be expressed in terms of the multipole moment. For an oscillating electric dipole of maximum value eR (Fig. 4.3a) the power radiated is

$$P_r = \frac{1}{4\pi\epsilon_0} \frac{\omega^4}{3c^3} (eR)^2 \quad \text{or} \quad \frac{1}{12\pi\epsilon_0} \frac{\omega^2 e^2}{c} \left(\frac{R}{\lambda}\right)^2 \qquad (4.17)$$

where ω and λ are the angular frequency and reduced wavelength respectively.

For an electric quadrupole of maximum value eR^2 (Fig. 4.3b) it is less than this by a factor of the order $(R/\lambda)^2$, and in general we can write

$$P_r \propto \left(\frac{R}{\lambda}\right)^{-2\ell} \qquad (4.18)$$

where $\ell = 1, 2$ etc., for dipole, quadrupole, etc. radiation.

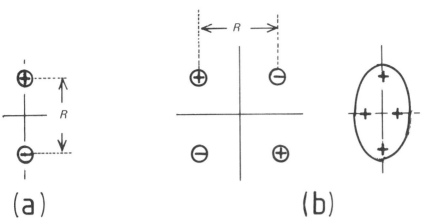

Fig. 4.3 (a) electric dipole; (b) electric quadrupoles

From consideration of typical values of R, which may be taken as the order of the nuclear diameter, and $\lambdabar$ the reduced wavelength of the γ-radiation, it is clear that higher multipole orders will have a lower probability per unit time for decay, and the corresponding nuclear states will have longer life-times. Typically $(R/\lambdabar)^2$ will be of order 10^{-4}. Although this is small, it does not prevent electric quadrupole transitions from being readily observed and frequently encountered in γ-decay. Somewhat similar generalisations can be made for magnetic transitions, which correspond to changes in the currents which circulate in the nucleus due to orbital motion of the protons, and the spins of neutrons and protons.

The multipolarity and character of a transition are related to change in spin and parity of the emitting nucleus. ΔI may take values $|I_f + I_i| > \Delta I > |I_f - I_i|$. Usually the smallest value $(I_f - I_i)$ is the most probable, but if a change of parity is involved (that is a change of symmetry of the wave-functions representing the nucleus), the probability is reduced, with a corresponding increase in the life-time of the state.

The electromagnetic interaction gives rise to life-times for γ-emission which are, in general, much shorter than the life-times for β-decay. Although a discussion of the techniques available for determining life-times of excited states is beyond the scope of this book, it should be said that coincidence techniques enable life-times down to 10^{-10} s to be measured, and that this limit can be further reduced by techniques using nuclear recoil and nuclear resonance fluorescence. A life-time which is sufficiently long to be measurable is called a **metastable state**, and a γ-transition from such a state is known as an **isomeric transition**. Occasionally transitions of high multipolarity are found for which the life-times are sufficiently long to be measured by radiochemical separation followed by direct measurement of activity as a function time. ^{119m}Sn and ^{137m}Ba (both with $\Delta I = 4$ and a change of parity) are examples of this, with half-lives of 250 d and 2.6 m respectively.

4.4 INTERNAL CONVERSION

The energy of an excited state of a nucleus can be transferred directly to an orbital electron which will then be ejected from the atom with a kinetic energy given by $E_\gamma - E_{K,L...}$, depending upon the shell from which the electron is ejected. Internal conversion therefore occurs as an alternative to the emission of gamma-radiation, and the ratio n_e/n_γ, where n_e and n_γ are respectively the numbers of conversion electrons and γ-photons emitted in unit time from

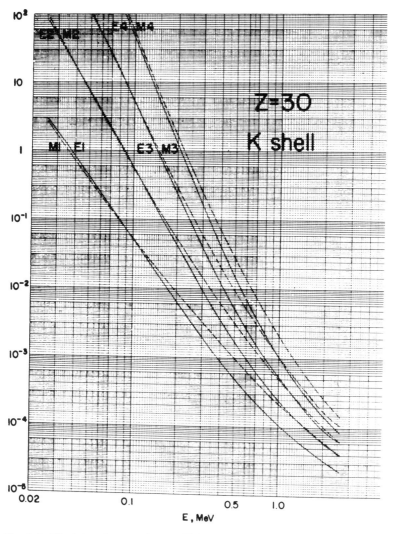

Fig. 4.4   The internal conversion coefficient, as a function of transition energy, for several different multipoles (Lederer *et al.*, 1966)

the radionuclide, is defined as the internal conversion coefficient, α. This may be subdivided into α_K, α_L, etc., for the various shells in which conversion takes place. The internal conversion coefficient will tend to be high in circumstances where the **radiative** probability is low, that is for transitions of high multipolarity and low energy. These features are illustrated in Fig. 4.4, taken from the compilation of Lederer *et al.* (1966).

Internal conversion is a single stage process, not involving an intermediate state of a γ-photon within the atom. This is conclusively demonstrated by experiments on technicium-99 m, in which the half-life of the isomeric transition has been found to be slightly dependent on the state of chemical combination of the technicium.

If internal conversion were a two-stage process, the life time would be determined by nuclear properties alone, and a change in $\psi^2(0)$ for an orbital electron, brought about by changing the state of chemical combination, would modify the internal conversion coefficient but would not affect the half-life.

In some radionuclides the probability of a γ-transition is so low that the decay of the isomeric state takes place entirely by the emission of conversion electrons, and observation of these is the only method by which the transition may be identified. In the special case of a $O^+ \rightarrow O^+$ transition, emission of γ-radiation is 'absolutely forbidden' and only internal conversion is possible. Examples of this are to be found in the spectrum of RaC[1] and ^{72}Ge.

Internal conversion electrons are directly observable as spectral lines superimposed on the continuous beta-spectrum. Their presence often needs to be taken note of in practical situations. For example, the internal dosimetry of radioisotopes must take account of conversion electrons, which will tend to deposit their energy within the medium, whereas γ-radiation emitted in the absence of internal conversion has a greater probability of emerging from the medium, thereby making a smaller contribution to the internal dose.

Internal conversion causes the appearance of a vacancy in one of the inner shells of the atom. This vacancy will be filled by an outer electron, causing the production of characteristic x-radiation, and this aspect is discussed in section 4.5 below.

4.5 *X*-RAYS FROM ELECTRON CAPTURE AND INTERNAL CONVERSION

We have seen that the inner shell vacancy produced by electron capture results in the production of x-rays characteristic of the $(Z - 1)$ element.

The electron capture process can be analysed by the Fermi statistical theory, and this aspect of the theoretical treatment is described by many authors for example Segrè (1977). It occurs with a probability proportional to the probability of the electron being found within the nuclear volume. This is essentially $\psi^2(0)$ for the electron wave function. Because the K shell orbit radius is proportional to Z^{-1}, the 'volume' occupied by the K electron is proportional to Z^{-3}, and the probability of finding the electron within the nuclear volume is thus proportional to Z^3. In fact, for an s wave function (applicable to electrons in the K, L_1, M_1, etc. shells)

$$\psi^2(0) = \frac{1}{\pi} \left(\frac{Z}{a_H}\right)^2 \cdot \frac{1}{n^3} \qquad (4.19)$$

where a_H is the Bohr hydrogen radius

$$a_H = \frac{1}{4\pi\epsilon_0} \frac{\hbar}{me^2} \qquad (4.20)$$

and n the principal quantum number, which is equal to 1 for the K shell.

The ratio of electron capture to positron emission (P_{EC}/P_+) therefore increases strongly with Z, partly because of the increasing probability of finding the electron within the nuclear volume, and partly because positron emission becomes progressively more inhibited on account of the increasing effect of the potential barrier as Z is increased.

The ratio is illustrated in Fig. 4.5, from which it can be seen that the emission of x-rays (or Auger electrons) becomes significant for Z greater than about 20.

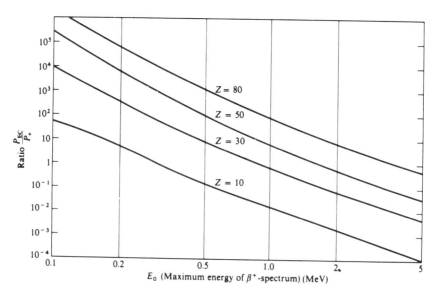

Fig. 4.5 Ratio of the probabilities of electron capture and positron emission, as a function of β^+ energy, for four different values of atomic number (after Feenberg and Trigg, 1950)

For $Q < E_K$, capture from the K shell is impossible, and only L capture can occur. The radioisotope ^{205}Pb would appear to be an example of this, although this particular feature of its decay does not seem to have been reported. For values of Q just slightly in excess of E_L the L spectrum predominates and the K spectrum is weak. This is the case in ^{235}Np. For Q values greatly in excess of E_K, the ratio P_L/P_K approaches a constant value of $1/8$, the ratio of the electron densities $\psi^2(0)$ for the 2 s subshell to the 1 s shell, each containing two electrons.

The subsequent filling of the K shell vacancy will result in the appearance of x-rays of the K spectrum of the daughter element, and also Auger electrons. The x-ray intensity is proportional to the fluorescence yield, which is given approximately by

$$\omega_K = \frac{Z^4}{a + Z^4} \tag{4.21}$$

where a is $\sim 1.1 \times 10^6$. Transitions of a non-radiative nature are possible, in which the transition energy appears as the kinetic energy of a second electron, leaving two vacancies in an atom which previously contained only one. These electrons are the Auger electrons, and consideration of (4.21), together with the binding energies of the relevant shells will show that the Auger electrons become less numerous, though substantially more energetic, as Z is increased. K x-rays and Auger electrons must be taken into consideration when evaluating the internal radiation dosimetry of K-capture radioisotopes (section 5.7).

Because the x-rays originate from a single vacancy, the relative intensities of the lines in the series are independent of the mode of production of the vacancy. The spectra observed in K-capture are therefore the same as those obtained by electron bombardment or X-ray fluorescence. The main lines in the spectrum are emitted during transitions between the energy levels for a singly-ionized atom, but there also occur some additional lines, of low intensity, known as satellites. These are usually due to double ionization of the KL type, in which vacancies appear simultaneously in the K and L shells. The relative probability of these second-order processes depends on the mode of vacancy production, but because of the low intensity of these satellite lines, they may be disregarded for many purposes, including dosimetry.

In the case of spectra in the L series, the line intensities do depend on the mode of vacancy production, and the relative ionization probabilities $L_1 : L_2 : L_3$ in orbital electron capture differ markedly from the values observed in other processes. L capture by itself is expected to be a somewhat rare process, because of the rather close constraints placed on the Q value of the decay $(E_L < Q < E_K)$, but, as we have seen, L capture in association with K capture occurs with significant probability. L capture occurs predominantly from the L_1 subshell, because of the greater value of $\psi^2(0)$ for this subshell as compared with the L_2 and L_3 subshells. This will be expected to increase the intensities of the lines of the L_1 sub-series above what is observed in the more conventional processes.

By far the greater number of L vacancies are produced as a consequence of the filling of the K shell, in the normal atomic processes of characteristic x-ray production, and so the relative intensity of L lines (and the ratio of L to K lines) produced in orbital electron capture will differ but little from the intensities listed by, for example Goldberg (1961) for electron bombardment. It should be emphasised however that this field has not been thoroughly explored, and that small differences may be expected to arise for the reasons given above.

The other principal mechanism for x-ray production is internal conversion. For conversion in the K-shell, the X-ray spectra are the same as expected from other processes, but for L conversion there are strong differences. The point is that in many radionuclides conversion in the L-shell occurs without K-conversion, so that the full differences between 'nuclear' and 'atomic' processes can be observed. Relative probabilities of $L_1:L_2:L_3$ conversion depend strongly on the character (magnetic or electric) and multipolarity of the nuclear transition, and therefore the relative intensities of the lines are also affected. For a magnetic dipole transition, conversion of the 2 s electrons (L_1 sub-shell) is more likely ($L_1:L_2:L_3 = 90:8:2$; Gellman et $al.$, 1950); whereas for an electric quadrupole transition ($\Delta I = 2$), ejection of the 2 p electrons (L_2 and L_3 subshells) is preferred ($L_1:L_2:L_3 = 3:55:42$). In the latter case, lines of the L_2 series (for example L_{β_1}, L_{γ_1}) are significantly stronger than are observed in electron emmission. Fig. 4.6 illustrates the L spectrum of uranium obtained by proton bombardment of a uranium salt and also by α-decay of ^{239}Pu. In the latter case (Fig. 4.6b) the L_{β_1} and L_{γ_1} lines are very strong compared with both the spectrum of Fig. 4.6a and the electron bombardment data of Goldberg.

Many heavy radionuclides emit L x-rays, following conversion (in the L shell) of low-energy gamma rays. An understanding of these is essential for accurate interpretation of X-ray spectra, and for dosimetry.

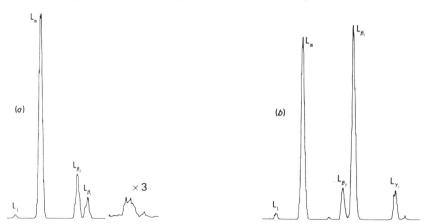

Fig. 4.6   L x-ray spectrum of uranium (a) 450 keV proton bombardment of uranyl acetate; (b) α-decay of plutonium–239 (Dyson, 1975)

4.6 POSITRON ANNIHILATION

When positrons are slowed down in matter, they eventually reach thermal velocities, and their cross-section for capture and annihilation with electrons becomes appreciable. The annihilation process converts the total mass-energy of the positron/electron pair, which is $2 m_0 c^2$ or approximately 1.02 MeV, into electromagnetic radiation. Assuming that momentum is conserved in the annihilation process and that this is zero, it is clear that at least two photons must be emitted. Two-photon annihilation is the most likely process, and accordingly we observed the emission of 2 photons of 0.511 MeV, emitted simultaneously in opposite directions. This radiation is a feature of the γ-spectrum observed from positron-emitting isotopes, because the positrons necessarily annihilate, if not within the source itself, then in adjacent shielding or other parts of the source mounting. The presence of annihilation radiation in the radiation from a source is a clear indication that decay is taking place by positron emission, at least in part.

An alternative mode of annihilation is that in which three photons are emitted. It may be shown that two-photon annihilation occurs when the positron and electron meet with spins opposed $(J = 0)$, whereas three-photon annihilation

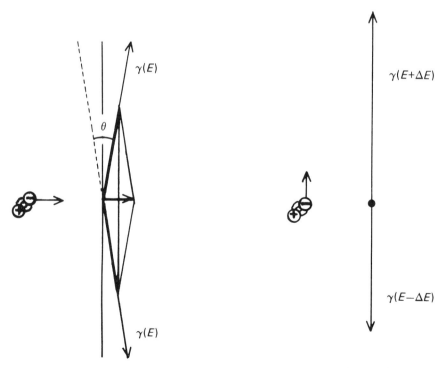

Fig. 4.7 Positron annihilation, with finite momentum of the annihilating electron

can only occur if the spins of the annihilating particles are aligned ($J = 1$). The conservation of linear momentum requires that, in the case of three-photon annihilation, the three photons be co-planner, but there is no restriction on the angles of emission, nor the energy of each photon, providing that the total is equal to 1.02 MeV. A weak continuous γ-ray spectrum is emitted in these circumstances. The annihilation probability in the 'spins-parallel' case is much smaller than for the 'spins-antiparallel' case (for example Segrè, 1977) and so in the circumstances outlined above, three-photon annihilation occurs in only a very small proportion (~ 1 in 10^3) of annihilations.

The assumption that the momentum of the annihilation pair is zero is not strictly true, because the energy of the electron may lie at any value between zero and the energy at the Fermi surface of the material in which annihilation is occurring. Let the 'Fermi energy' be denoted by E_f. If we make the simple assumption that the maximum momentum, p, is given by $\sqrt{2mE_f}$, we see from Fig. 4.8 that the photons will be emitted in a cone of semi-angle ϕ, which is of the order

$$\frac{pc}{E_\gamma} = \frac{\sqrt{2mE_f}}{mc} = \sqrt{\frac{2E_f}{mc^2}} \tag{4.22}$$

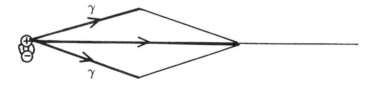

Fig. 4.8 Annihilation in flight

If E_f is taken as ~ 5 eV, this is of the order of 15 milliradians. Furthermore, the net motion of the annihilating pair will impose a Doppler shift upon the annihilation radiation which will extend up to a displacement (from mc^2) which is of order

$$\Delta E = \frac{v}{c} mc^2 = pc, \quad \text{or} \quad (2mE_f)^{\frac{1}{2}}.c \tag{4.23}$$

which is of the order of 2 keV. This is observable as a line broadening if a Ge(Li) detector of good resolution is used for the measurements, and if there are unbroadened 'nuclear' γ-rays in the same part of the spectrum for comparison.

If the position is being slowed down, there is a finite probability that annihilation with electrons in the slowing-down medium will take place before thermal velocities are reached. This 'annihilation in flight' will necessarily cause the annihilation radiation to be directed in the forward hemisphere, in order to conserve momentum, and the energy of the electromagnetic radiation will exceed $2\,m_0c^2$ because of the kinetic energy possessed by the positron.

When positrons have reached thermal velocities, a bound state can in some circumstances be formed with an electron prior to annihilation. This neutral system has some of the characteristics of an atom, and is known as positronium. It exists in two states – singlet (para) and triplet (ortho) positronium. These states are formed in ratios corresponding to their multiplicities $(2\,J + 1)$, that is in the ratio of $1:3$. Three-quarters of positronium atoms are therefore formed in the triplet state.

The triplet state annihilates by the three-quantum processes, so it is clear that, in circumstances where positronium is formed, the likelihood of three-photon annihilation can be much greater than when annihilation takes place between unbound positrons and electrons. The life times of singlet and triplet positronium are of the order of 10^{-10} s and 10^{-7} s respectively. The triplet positronium can survive the time to annihilation only if the probability of losing the aligned spins by collision ('quenching') is small. Quenching is least probable in certain organic gases, notably halogen-substituted hydrocarbons such as difluorodichloromethane (CF_2Cl_2), (in which a 'collision complex', $e^+CCl_2F_2$ is formed), but occurs readily in the presence of gas molecules which have unpaired spins (for example NO) or which possess an atomic magnetic field (for example O_2).

4.7 THE ABSOLUTE ACTIVITY OF RADIOACTIVE SOURCES

Although it is not the place of this book to give an account of the many instrumental techniques available for the study of nuclear decay schemes, one aspect of radioactive sources is of particular importance in the medical context, and that is its **Activity**, or number of disintegrations taking place per unit time in the source. An additional important feature of a source is the **γ-ray dose rate** at a given distance from the source. These two quantities may be combined into the **specific gamma emission**, which is the dose rate (at a given distance) per unit of activity. Knowledge of this quantity is important whenever a radioactive source is used for external irradiation of a chemical or biological system, and is also important in the context of radiation protection.

The unit of Activity in common use is the Curie, which is defined as 3.700×10^{10} disintegrations per second of a named isotope. When this unit came into existence it was defined as the activity of 1 **gram of radium**. Technical difficulties in the measurement of disintegration rate of this particular material meant that the physical realisation of this unit could never be accurate to better than about 1 percent, and so the unit was redefined in accordance with the exact definition given here.

In the case of radioisotopes which decay into active daughter products, this definition can still be applied. For example, 1 Curie of ^{90}Sr will 'generate' 1 Curie of the daughter ^{90}Y, and a correct description of such a source would be '1 Curie of ^{90}Sr in equilibrium with 1 Curie of ^{90}Y'.

The Curie is being superseded by the S.I. unit of Activity, the **Becquerel**, which is defined as 1 disintegration per second, of a named radionuclide.

4.7.1 β^--emitters

The simplest method of measuring the activity of a β-emitter is to set up a 'defined solid angle' experiment as illustrated in Fig. 4.9. An end-window Geiger counter is suitable for this purpose, as its efficiency for most β-emitters is close to 100%. Clearly the counting rate N_β in such a system will be given by

$$N_\beta = N \frac{\omega}{4\pi} \tag{4.24}$$

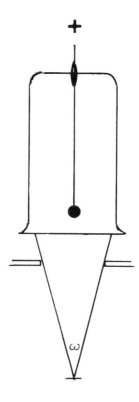

Fig. 4.9 'Defined solid angle' method for determining the disintegration rate of a β^--emitter

Several fundamental shortcomings of this method should be noted.

(1) The effective solid angle cannot always be measured with great accuracy.

(2) There is always the possibility that the β-particles at the extreme low energy end of the spectrum will be absorbed in the counter window. One way of allowing for this effect is to place absorbers of several known thicknesses in front of the window, and extrapolate the counting-rate to zero thickness. The window thickness will usually be known, so that this procedure can be carried out in practice. There must always be some error, however, associated with such a procedure, on account of the uncertainties inherent in the extrapolation process.

(3) If some of the β decays proceed to excited states of (stable) daughter nucleus, there will be gamma radiation emitted, and this can in principle contribute to the total observed counting rate. This effect is small because the efficiency of a Geiger counter for γ-radiation is usually small, of the order of 1%.

(4) If some of the γ-rays are internally converted, the conversion electrons will be counted with high efficiency, and will introduce serious error. This method is therefore only applicable if internal conversion is known not to occur in the isotope under investigation.

A more satisfactory procedure is to use the 4π-counter illustrated in Fig. 4.10. This consists of 2 hemispheres, each with its own anode collecting wire. They are fitted together, with the source material deposited on a thin plastic film and mounted inside. The counter can then be filled with the correct gas mixture, normally using a continuous flow system. Although such a counter could, in principle, be operated in the Geiger region it is more usual to operate it as a proportional counter; much higher counting rates can be employed, because of the short dead time, and some pulse discrimination can be used if necessary.

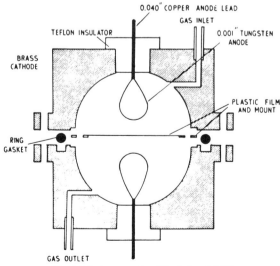

Fig. 4.10 4π-counter (Siegbahn, 1965)

The 4π-counter is free from all the disadvantages listed above – the presence of associated γ-radiation will not make an independent contribution to the counting rate because the γ-photons will normally be simultaneous with the β-particles and will not create an independent event, unless the γ-ray proceeds from a metastable state. Internal conversion similarly will not normally increase the counting rate, furthermore, there will be no losses of the kind associated with the passage of the β-particles through a counter window, and if a suitably thin source is prepared, self-absorption effects are very small.

The methods just described are based on the assumption that the counting efficiency is 100%, but this assumption can be avoided if there is a γ-photon associated with each β-particle. Consider the arrangement shown in Fig. 4.11, and let us examine the possibility of counts being produced simultaneously in both the β and γ-channels. Such events can be detected by suitable coincidence circuits, and expressions for the counting rates can be set up as follows.

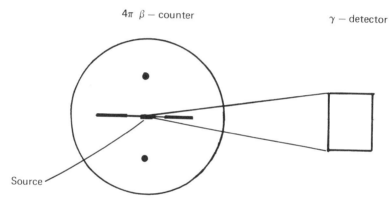

Fig. 4.11 $4\pi\beta$-counter in coincidence with a γ-ray detector

Let N_β and N_γ be the counting rates (assumed to have been corrected for counting losses) in the β and γ channels.

Then $N_\beta = N_0 \epsilon_\beta$

The number of coincident $(\beta\gamma)$ events per unit time is given by

$$N_{\beta\gamma} = N_0 \epsilon_\beta \epsilon_\gamma$$

where ϵ_γ is the efficiency of the γ detectors (the quantity ϵ_γ is taken to include also the solid angle terms of the form $\omega/4\pi$).

Furthermore,

$$N_\gamma = N_0 \epsilon_\gamma$$

Hence, combining these equations we obtain

$$\epsilon_\gamma = \frac{N_{\beta\gamma}}{N_\beta} \; ; \; \epsilon_\beta = \frac{N_{\beta\gamma}}{N_\gamma} \; ; \; \text{and}$$

$$N_0 = \frac{N_\beta N_\gamma}{N_{\beta\gamma}} \tag{4.25}$$

We thus have a reliable method of obtaining the absolute activity of a sample.

If not all the β-particles are in coincidence with a γ-photon, but only a fraction f, the equations become

$$N_\beta = N_0 \epsilon_\beta \; ; \; N_{\beta\gamma} = N_0 \epsilon_\beta (1 - f)\epsilon_\gamma$$

and $$N_\gamma = N_0 f \epsilon_\gamma$$

Hence $$N_0 = \frac{N_\beta N_\gamma}{N_{\beta\gamma}} \cdot \frac{1-f}{f}, \tag{4.26}$$

and the absolute activity cannot be determined unless the fraction f is known.

If the β-counter has a small detection efficiency for γ-radiation, we may proceed as follows (confining ourselves to the case where *all* β-particles have an associated coincident γ-photon).

$$N_\beta = N_0 \epsilon_\beta + N_0 (1 - \epsilon_\beta)\epsilon_{\beta\gamma}$$

$$N_{\beta\gamma} = N_0 \epsilon_\beta \epsilon_\gamma \; ; \; N_\gamma = N_0 \epsilon_\gamma$$

where $\epsilon_{\beta\gamma}$ is the detection efficiency of the β-counter for γ-radiation.

Hence $$\frac{N_\beta N_\gamma}{N_{\beta\gamma}} = N_0 (1 - \frac{(1 - \epsilon_\beta)}{\epsilon_\beta} \cdot \epsilon_{\beta\gamma})$$

If ϵ_β is varied (for example by interposing thin foils between source and detector) a graph of the kind shown in Fig. 4.12 may be plotted, from which N_0 may be obtained by extrapolating to $\frac{1 - \epsilon_\beta}{\epsilon_\beta} = 0$. The occurrence of internal conversion will effectively increase the quantity $\epsilon_{\beta\gamma}$ and will therefore alter the gradient of the graph plotted in Fig. 4.12, but will not alter the result of the extrapolation procedure.

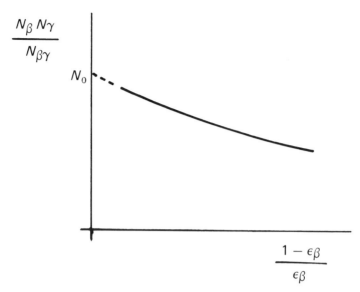

Fig. 4.12 Determination of absolute activity (see text)

4.7.2 2 γ-photons in cascade

This situation applies in the important case of ^{60}Co. The coincidence method (here used to examine coincidences between 2 gamma-photons) yields the result

$$N = \frac{N_{\gamma_1} N_{\gamma_2}}{N_{\gamma\gamma}} \tag{4.27}$$

where N_{γ_1} and N_{γ_2} are the rates in the two counting channels and $N_{\gamma\gamma}$ is the coincidence counting rate. Note again that the result is independent of the efficiency of the two detectors, and hence, by implication, independent of the solid angles subtended by the two detectors.

4.7.3 Electron capture and β^+ emitters

A 4π-counter of the type illustrated in Fig. 4.10 is also suitable for the detection of positrons, and can therefore be used for neutron-deficient isotopes which emit positrons, or for those odd-odd radionuclides which decay both by β^- and β^+ emission. However, a problem arises because of the electron capture processes which normally occur as alternatives to positron emission. The x-rays emitted following electron capture may escape from the detector, although Auger electrons will be stopped, and therefore recorded, because of their short range. To detect the X-rays, a counter of relatively large dimensions filled with a gas of moderately high atomic number is suitable. Readings are normally taken at several different pressures, and the counting rate obtained by extrapolation to

$1/p \to 0$ is a reliable measure of the source activity. An internal source is required to avoid loss of x-rays or Auger electrons by absorption in the counter windows. If the x-ray energy is low, a single pressure will suffice, and the radionuclide may be incorporated into the counter gas, providing that the mean free path of the x-rays is small compared with the counter dimensions. If the atomic number of the radionuclide is small or moderate, there will be the further advantage that the fluorescence yield is low. Most of the decay processes will then produce Auger electrons, which are of short range.

4.8 EXTERNAL DOSIMETRY OF RADIATION SOURCES

4.8.1 α-sources;

Sources of α-particles are not often used as external sources in radiobiological work, and never in medical applications. The range of α-particles (40 μm for a 4 MeV α-particle in soft tissue) is too small to be of value in the medical field, although in radiobiology α-particle beams could, in principle, be used for irradiation of tissue cultures or other preparations, providing their thickness does not exceed the dimensions of a single biological cell. However, α-particles are made use of in related fields, such as thermoluminescence research, and so a knowledge of external α-particle dosimetry is occasionally required.

The dosimetry of α-particles is best evaluated from a knowledge of the specific energy-loss in the medium of interest. This quantity $(\mathrm{d}E/\mathrm{d}(\rho x)$, as discussed in section 1.3) is well-documented (for example Williamson *et al.*, 1966) for many elements, having been obtained from calculations based on the Bethe–Bloch formula, with corrections derived from experimental data.

To obtain the specific energy-loss for non-elemental materials, the atomic composition needs to be known, and the combined effect of the constituent elements can be obtained additively. This means essentially that we can write

$$\frac{\mathrm{d}E}{\mathrm{d}(\rho x)} = \left(\frac{\mathrm{d}E}{\mathrm{d}(\rho x)}\right)_1 w_1 + \left(\frac{\mathrm{d}E}{\mathrm{d}(\rho x)}\right)_2 w_2 + \dots \tag{4.28}$$

where the subscripts $1, 2 \dots$ refer to the different elements present in the material, and $w_1, w_2 \dots$ are the proportions by weight of each element.

The flux of α-particles can be measured by particle-detection methods, and the radiation dose obtained by direct calculation of the absorbed energy per unit mass.

Some secondary electrons will be projected away from the immediate vicinity of the α-particle tracks. These are the δ-rays which are referred to in section 1.2. The maximum energy E_e of a free electron 'knocked-on' by a heavy particle of energy E_0 is given by

$$E_e = \frac{4m}{m} E_0 \tag{4.29}$$

where m, M are the masses of the light and heavy particles respectively. For a 4 MeV α-particle this works out to be approximately 2 keV. The range of these is only in the region of $0.2\,\mu\text{m}$ in material with the density of water. Even the thinnest sample for irradiation of biological or other material would have a thickness greater than this. Escape of the δ-rays can therefore be neglected, and all may be assumed to make their due contribution to the radiation dose received by the sample. In a small proportion of interactions, greater energy transfers, producing longer δ-ray tracks, are possible.

Although the energy in the form of δ-rays is unlikely to leave the system being irradiated, it should be noted that the distribution of energy on the microscopic (cellular) scale is of considerable importance when considering the biological effects of radiation at the cellular level. In particular, we distinguish between the densely-ionizing track formed by the α-particle itself, and the more lightly-ionizing tracks caused by the δ-rays. The relative proportion of energy deposited in these two forms is a significant determinant of biological effect, and this aspect of the dosimetry of densely-ionizing radiation is referred to again in section 6.1.

4.8.2 β-sources

β-particles from radioactive sources have ranges which may approach 1 cm in water or biological tissue, and so are frequently used in radiobiological work. Their use in clinical medicine has been established for many years, for example in the treatment of small lesions of the cornea of the eye using β-ray 'applicators' to deliver the required radiation dose; and, more recently, in the technique of electron therapy using beams with an energy of several MeV extracted from linear accelerators. For dosimetric purposes, calculations based on the known specific energy-loss are not satisfactory because of the substantial amount of scattering which occurs in the beam – the amount of energy deposited by an electron requires integration of the specific energy-loss along the whole track,

$$E_2 - E_1 = \int_{\text{initial}}^{\text{final}} \frac{\mathrm{d}E}{\mathrm{d}x}\,\mathrm{d}x \tag{4.30}$$

which may significantly exceed the actual thickness of the material being irradiated. The error will be greatest in high Z materials where the scattering is greatest, but even in low Z materials the scattering readily occurs, as revealed in cloud chamber or nuclear emulsion photographs of β-particle tracks. Experimental determinations are therefore important, and small thin-walled ionization chambers have been devised for β-particle dosimetry. In effect, the dose in air may be established, and then converted to doses in water or tissue, knowing the relative stopping powers for the two media.

The dose rate from a point source of β-particles has been expressed by many authors as

$$D_\beta = K e^{-\nu x} (\nu x)^{-2} \qquad (4.31)$$

In this expression $e^{-\nu x}$ expresses the fact that the counting rate from a β-particle source is often obtained to vary approximately exponentially with the thickness of air, or other material, intervening between source and detector. An effective 'attenuation coefficient', ν, for the intervening medium, may be introduced to represent this functional dependence, and has been found useful in dosimetric work. The term $(\nu x)^{-2}$ represents the ordinary inverse square law. K depends upon the β-ray energy, the source activity, and the material being irradiated.

Once a point source distribution function has been established, it may be used to calculate the dose rate from sources of other sizes, for example line sources, or sources distributed over two dimensions. These extensions introduce no new physical principles, and for details the specialist literature must be consulted, for example Attix, Roesch and Tochilin (1969) or Spiers (1968).

We shall see in section 5.9 how this approach can also be applied to dose rates from β-emitters which are distributed within the material, or tissue, undergoing irradiation.

4.8.3 γ-sources

Calculation of 'exposure' and absorbed doses for point sources of γ-emitters is based on a knowledge of the mass energy-absorption coefficients in air and in other media. An important quantity in this connection is the 'specific γ-emission' (Γ) of a radionuclide. This may be expressed in terms of exposure, dose rate in air or dose rate in tissue. It is defined in roentgens (or rads in air or in tissue) per unit time and per unit of activity, at a stipulated distance (usually one metre) from a point source, neglecting any absorption in the source or in the intervening air. A simple calculation will make this clear.

Suppose that a source emits one photon per disintegration and that there is no internal conversion. For a disintegration rate of N we may write, for the dose-rate in air at a distance r.

$$D_\gamma = \frac{N E_\gamma}{4\pi r^2} (\mu/\rho)_{\text{air}} \qquad (4.32)$$

where $(\mu/\rho)_{\text{air}}$ is the mass energy-absorption coefficient and E_γ the photon energy. If E_γ is in Joules, r in centimetres and (μ/ρ) in $(\text{cm})^2\,\text{g}^{-1}$, D_γ will be given in Joule $(gm)^{-1} s^{-1}$. To obtain Γ in rads (in air) $mCi^{-1} h^{-1}$ at 1 metre, and expressing E_γ in MeV, we may write

$$\Gamma = \frac{E_\gamma}{4\pi\, 10^4}(\mu/\rho)_{air} \times 3.7 \times 10^7 \times 3600 \times 10^5 \times 1.602 \times 10^{-13}$$

$$= E_\gamma(\mu/\rho)_{air}\, 1.698 \times 10^{-2} \text{ rad } hr^{-1}\, mCi^{-1} @ 1 \text{ metre.} \qquad (4.33)$$

For $E_\gamma = 1$ MeV $(\mu/\rho)_{air}$ is 0.28 $(cm)^2\, g^{-1}$,

hence $\Gamma = 4.76 \times 10^{-3}$ air rads $(mCi)^{-1} h^{-1}$ at 1 metre;

or 5.48×10^{-3} roentgen $(mCi)^{-1} h^{-1}$ at 1 metre

or 5.2×10^{-3} tissue rads $(mCi)^{-1} h^{-1}$ at 1 metre,

using the conversion factors given in section 3.5.

These data are frequently expressed in graphical form, as shown in Fig. 4.13. If a decay scheme is known, the specific gamma emission can be calculated by a simple addition of the contribution from the several γ-rays emitted, taking care to allow for any internal conversion of these. Emitted x-rays also contribute to the specific gamma emission, although these are best expressed separately, in view of the likelihood of their being absorbed, in any practical situation, by relatively small thicknesses of material.

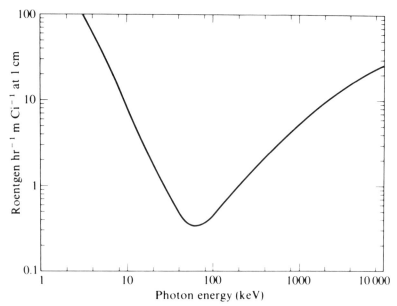

Fig. 4.13 Specific γ-emission as a function of photon energy, assuming 1 photon per disintegration (Dyson, 1973)

As in the case of β-radiation, the point source function can be used to calculate the radiation dose from line sources or other 2-dimensional distributions. For γ-radiation the point source function is fundamental in nature, and can be used with good accuracy and reliability for this procedure.

In both cases, the calculation gives the absorbed dose at the surface of a medium only. In order to calculate dose rates beneath the surface, more elaborate procedures are needed, and the determination of dose rate is then best achieved by experimental procedures. Much work has been carried out, using ionization chambers immersed in a suitable medium (usually water), to investigate the depth dose distribution of radiation from collimated beams of γ-radiation from strong radioisotope sources of ^{60}Co and ^{137}Cs which are used extensively for practical applications in radiobiology and medical physics.

In the case of a narrow beam of radiation the photons which interact by any of the processes described in Chapter 1 will be either totally absorbed, or scattered out of the beam. The intensity of monoenergetic radiation will therefore fall exponentially with depth and can be calculated from the known mass attenuation coefficients of the material comprising the medium. At the photon energies of ^{60}Co and ^{137}Cs the Compton cross-section for back-scattering is relatively small and so will not contribute significantly to the dose at a given point along the narrow beam in the medium.

However, beams used for practical purposes in medical and radiation physics, are not narrow, and so there is an appreciable contribution, at points on the axis, from radiation scattered-in from peripheral points of the beam. This is illustrated in Fig. 4.14 where the 'depth dose distributions' for different field sizes are

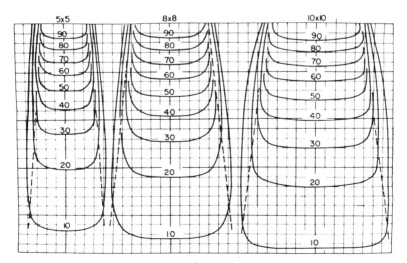

Fig. 4.14   Depth-dose distribution for ^{137}Cs radiation, for square fields of 3 different sizes. Distance from source to surface of medium 35 cm (after Johns, 1964) (By courtesy of Charles C. Thomas, Publisher, Springfield, Illinois.)

illustrated for the radiation from ^{137}Cs. The wider beams give somewhat greater doses at a given depth, and the differences between field sizes is more pronounced the greater the depth within the medium.

The effect of varying the photon energy, for a given field size, is shown in Fig. 4.15. The 'harder' radiation shows a greater degree of penetration, bringing obvious advantages for the treatment of deep seated tumors by radiotherapy. The presence of scattered radiation outside the beam may also be noted. This is less pronounced for the ^{60}Co radiation than for ^{137}Cs because of the increasing tendency of Compton scattering to be in the **forward** direction as the photon energy is increased. For comparison a set of data for x-radiation generated at 250 kV from a tungsten target is shown. The penetration is less than for the higher energy sources, and the side-scatter is much greater than in the case of ^{60}Co radiation, though not greatly different from ^{137}Cs.

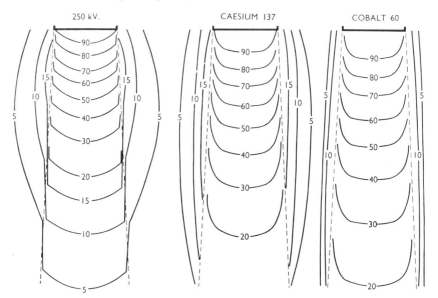

Fig. 4.15   Depth-dose distributions for different radiations. Field size 5 cm × 5 cm
(Meredith and Massey, 1969)

It may be noted that ionization dosimetry affords a convenient method of determining source activity, if the material has a known decay scheme and is radioisotopically pure. 'Re-entrant' ionization chambers (Fig. 4.16) are in use for this type of work. The chamber may be designed so that it is relatively insensitive to variation in the position, shape or size of the source placed inside. It may then be used on a routine basis for monitoring cyclotron targets, radio-chemically separated material, or radioisotopes being dispensed for practical use. A re-entrant chamber has to be calibrated with standards of each radioisotope for which it is to be used.

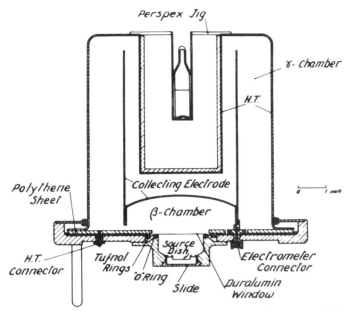

Fig. 4.16 Re-entrant ionization chamber (Dale *et al.*, 1961)

FURTHER READING

Attix, F. H., Roesch, W. C. and Tochilin, E. (Eds.) (1969) *Radiation Dosimetry*
    3 volumes Academic Press
Dyson, N. A. (1973) *X-rays in atomic and nuclear physics* Longman

REFERENCES

Becker, R. (1964) *Electromagnetic Fields and Interactions* Blackie
Dale, J. W. G., Perry, W. E. and Pulfer, R. F. (1961) *Int. Journ. App. Rad. and
    Isotopes,* **10**, 65
Dyson, N. A. (1975) *Phys. Med. Biol.,* **20**, 1
Evans, R. D. (1955) See Further Reading for Chapter 1
Feenberg, E. and Trigg, G. (1950) *Rev. Mod. Phys.* **22**, 399
Goldberg, M. (1961) *J. Phys. Radium,* **22**, 743
Johns, H. E. (1964) *The Physics of Radiology* Thomas
Lederer, C. M., Hollander, J. M., Perlman, I. (1966) *Table of Isotopes* Wiley
Meredith, W. J. and Massey, J. B. (1969) *Fundamental Physics of Radiology*
    Williams and Wilkins, Baltimore
Segrè (1977) See Further Reading for Chapter 1
Siegbahn (1965) See Further Reading for Chapter 3
Spiers, F. W. (1968) See References for Chapter 3
Williamson, C. F., *et al.* (1966) See References for Chapter 1

CHAPTER 5

Applications of Radioisotopes in Medicine and Biology

5.1 INTRODUCTION – GENERAL BEHAVIOUR OF RADIOISOTOPES IN THE BODY

Living organisms depend for survival upon a complex interplay of physical and biochemical processes, in order to fulfill essential functions such as nutrition, excretion, respiration, etc. Elements and ionic species participate in these processes by virtue of their physical and chemical properties, in determining, for example, the rate at which a diffusion process or a chemical reaction takes place; methods of pursuing an element along its 'metabolic pathway' are clearly of fundamental importance in the study of life processes. The existence of radio-isotopes is of great importance in such studies – radioactive ions or molecules can be introduced into the system, or existing molecules can be 'labelled' by substituting one or more atoms with radioactive isotopes of those elements, and their route within and through the system can then be followed by the many techniques available for the detection of the emitted radiations. This use of radio-isotopes as 'tracers' has contributed greatly to our understanding of biochemical processes. It is not essential that a tracer be radioactive. Stable isotopes can in principle be used, and are of practical value in a few rather special situations; but methods of measuring (stable) isotopic composition are technically difficult to apply and rarely useful in the practical context, the main area of application being the possibility of labelling water with the heavy isotope deuterium (in the form of heavy water, D_2O), whose chemical and physical properties are sufficiently different from ordinary water to enable isotopic composition to be determined by, for example, the measurements of density. Furthermore, a tracer can some-times consist of a different element, for instance Br^- to trace the behaviour of Cl^-, which in some respects it resembles; and again, coloured dyes have been used to reveal the flow paths, and also the dilution factors, of body fluids. But the radioactive tracer remains of primary importance in this field, and this chapter will be concerned essentially with radioactive isotopes.

As a result of being able to study physiological function by tracer techniques, it is possible to establish limits of normal function, and to use this information as a basis for diagnostic tests in clinical medicine. The normal and also the pathological behaviour of iodine in the body, for example, has been studied in detail, enabling its particular role to be understood quantitatively (section 5.5).

From the foregoing description of the potential uses of radioisotopes, it is clearly essential to ensure that the radiation doses delivered to any part of the body are insufficient to modify cellular function in any way. But by administering a sufficiently large amount of a radioisotope, the radiation dose can be sufficient to cause a modification of function, and this has given rise to radioisotope therapy using for example ^{32}P for the treatment of **polycythaemia**, or isotopes of iodine for the treatment of **thyrotoxicosis** (section 5.7).

To describe the behaviour of radioisotopes in the body, we speak of the 'space' for that particular ionic or molecular species. This essentially qualitative concept describes the appropriate subdivision of the body to which it has access. In cases where the ion is confined to one or other of the fluid spaces of the body (for example extracellular or intracellular fluid) the 'space' can be described more quantitatively in terms of an effective fluid volume. We speak of the 'sodium space', 'potassium space', and so on.

'Spaces' are subdivided into **compartments**, the latter being a volume throughout which an ion or molecule can diffuse freely compared with its entry into (or exit from) other volumes. This may be free mixing throughout a liquid (for instance plasma), or diffusion through various fluids in the body. A compartment has been well-described (Matthews, 1971) as "an anatomical, physiological, chemical or physical subdivision of the substance considered". Or, in certain cases, a compartment may be the whole of the 'space' for the substance, the best-known example of this situation being that of total body water — if a molecule of water is introduced into the body, by whatever route, it has free access to all fluid compartments in the body — extracellular (including plasma), intracellular, and, 'transcellular' (for example the cerebro-spinal fluid).

Although the 'space' is essentially a qualitative concept, it can become quantitative when the amount of material actually present is considered. The total amount of an element (or ion) is referred to as the 'pool' of that substance, and the total amount is referred to as the **pool mass**. We shall see that the pool mass (as well as the compartment **volumes** referred to earlier) can be determined by tracer methods.

5.2 DETERMINATION OF COMPARTMENT VOLUMES AND POOL MASSES BY THE ISOTOPE DILUTION METHOD

If a compartment is isolated, in the sense that transport to or from other compartments can take place only very slowly if at all, this technique is applicable. If an activity Q of a suitable label is introduced into a volume V, we can write

$Q = VC$,   where C is the concentration, or activity per unit volume.

If this is now added to a volume V' and mixed, we can write

$$Q = C'(V + V'), \quad \text{where } C' \text{ is the new concentration.}$$

$$\therefore \ V' = V\left(\frac{C}{C'} - 1\right)$$

or, if $\quad V' \gg V$,

$$V' = V\frac{C}{C'} \tag{5.1}$$

The volume V' may thus be determined by measuring the ratio of the concentrations C/C'. This is known as the isotope dilution method, and is valid if complete mixing, or **equilibration**, occurs, in which the ratio of tracer atoms to ordinary atoms is the same in all regions of the compartment.

A simple example will suffice. To determine the volume of water in the body (or total body water) a known volume of water labelled with the radioisotope tritium is introduced, for example by oral administration. The activity need not be known in absolute terms, but the counting rate from a standard volume introduced into a counting system of fixed geometry must be known.

Samples of water are then obtained, at intervals, over a few hours, from plasma or urine, and the activity per unit volume in this will be seen to reach an equilibrium value after a few hours, from which the volume of total body water may be calculated from (5.1). Because C and C' may differ by a factor of the order of 1000, it is normal to prepare a standard which is diluted by a known factor, so that the counting system is being used for comparing concentrations which do not differ by a very large factor.

By this method the volume of total body water is found to be about 45 litres. If the subject is avoiding fluid intake, but losing water gradually in the perspiration or urine, this will not affect the activity per unit volume of fluid, because the fluid lost will also have the same activity per unit volume. The value for total body water found by this method is that at the time of equilibration. To allow for loss before equilibration, (5.1) must be corrected by writing

$$V' = \frac{Q - q}{C'} \tag{5.2}$$

where q is the activity lost during the equilibration period.

We have noted earlier that, from the point of view of a molecule of water, the water in the body forms a single compartment. For some ions, however, we must distinguish between various compartments within the total body water. In particular, we distinguish between the extracellular fluid ($\sim$20 litres) and the intracellular fluid ($\sim$25 litres). The extracellular fluid includes interstitial water,

water in connective tissue, plasma, and also the 'transcellular' water, that is, water which has traversed cells, but is not contained within cells, for example the cerebrospinal fluid and the aqueous humour of the eye. To determine the extra-cellular and intracellular compartment volumes, different tracers are required. For example, the bromide ion Br^- remains essentially in the extracellular fluid, whereas potassium, as K^+ ions, is found predominantly in the intracellular fluid. The extracellular fluid volume may be determined by applying the isotope dilution method, using Br^- as a tracer, and the intracellular fluid then found by difference. Further discussion of these fluid compartments is to be found in section 5.4.

A further type of measurement is the determination of the amount (that is, the mass) of an ion or molecule in a given compartment. The isotope dilution method may be applied to this, by introducing a known activity into the system, and then determining the **specific activity** (that is activity per unit mass) of the tracer after equilibration has taken place. Chemical assay is therefore required, to determine the mass of material present in the sample. The absolute activity is not required, and the counting rates in a 'fixed geometry' counting system are normally the quantities determined.

Electrolytes such as Na^+ can be studied by this method, although it should be noted that, in this case, the tracer will not at any stage become uniformly distributed throughout the total body sodium. Parts of the skeletal sodium are relatively inaccessible ('non-exchangeable') and will not be include in determina-tions carried out by this method (for example after 24 hours equilibration time), which is accordingly confined to the exchangeable sodium only. It should further be noted that, although the exchangeable sodium is found mainly in the extracellular fluid, it is not confined there; the apparent compartment **volume** (apparent sodium space) determined by this method is in fact appreciably greater than the extracellular fluid volume (27.8 litres as compared with about 20 litres) and does not correspond to any physically identifiable volume, although a comparison between these two volumes is an indication of the extent to which exchangeable sodium moves out into other compartments, in this case into the intracellular fluid and the exchangeable fraction of sodium in bone.

Having established some definitions, and noted in passing some of the approximations and limitations which have to be borne in mind when measuring compartment volumes and pool masses, we are now in a position to analyse the dynamic behaviour of tracers in the body and to set up models describing this.

5.3 COMPARTMENT THEORY

The discussion in the previous section supposed that we were dealing with a 'closed' system or at least that the system can be regarded as closed for the duration of the measurement. In practice we are concerned with an 'open' system, at equilibrium in the sense that the concentrations of electrolytes and molecular substances are in a steady state. To take the simplest case of a **single compartment open system**, (Fig. 5.1) suppose that m atoms (ions, molecules)

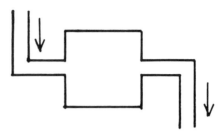

Fig. 5.1 A single compartment open system

per unit time be added to a system at equilibrium containing M atoms of the same substance. We defined a turnover rate, K, equal to m/M. Now suppose that x tracer atoms are present. If these behave in the same way as the substance being traced, we can write

$$\frac{\mathrm{d}x/\mathrm{d}t}{x} = -K,$$

and this differential equation represents the behaviour of the system. If x_0 atoms of tracer are introduced as a single administration at $t = 0$, we see readily that the solution of the equation is

$$x = x_0 e^{-Kt}.$$

If the tracer is a radioisotope with decay constant λ.

$$\frac{\mathrm{d}x}{\mathrm{d}t} = -Kx - \lambda x \qquad (5.3)$$

Hence $x = x_0 e^{-(K+\lambda)t}$

The system is characterised by an exponential decay, and we define the biological half-life (τ_b) of the substance as $\dfrac{\ln 2}{K}$. The radioactive half-life (τ_r) is of course $\dfrac{\ln 2}{\lambda}$, and we can define the **effective half-life** (τ_{eff}) as $\dfrac{\ln 2}{K+\lambda}$ or

$$\frac{1}{\tau_{\mathrm{eff}}} = \frac{1}{\tau_b} + \frac{1}{\tau_r}.$$

Total body water behaves in this way, and has a biological half-life in the region of 12 days.

Now consider a continuous input of radioactive atoms per unit time, R.

We can write $\quad dx/dt = -(K + \lambda)x + R$

Hence $\qquad x = \dfrac{R(1 - e^{-(K + \lambda)t})}{K + \lambda}$ \hfill (5.4)

showing that the activity $(=x\lambda)$ rises to an equilibrium value of $\dfrac{R}{K + \lambda}$ after a sufficiently long time. Note that if the turnover rate is small, the activity in the system will take a long time to build up, but will tend towards a larger final value than otherwise.

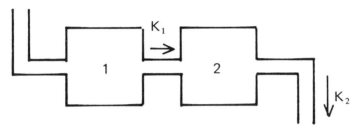

Fig. 5.2 A two-compartment open system

The **two-compartment open system** (Fig. 5.2) can be analysed as follows: Let the turnover rate in compartment 1 (that is the fraction of molecules leaving – or entering – compartment 1 per unit time) be K_1. We make the assumption that the flow is in the direction shown by the arrows in Fig. 5.2 and that there is no back-diffusion from compartment 2 into compartment 1.

Hence $\qquad \dfrac{dx_1/dt}{x_1} = -(K_1 + \lambda)$ \hfill (5.5)

In compartment 2, $\dfrac{dx_2}{dx} = -(\lambda + K_2)x_2 + K_1 x_1$ \hfill (5.6)

where the turnover rate in compartment 2 is K_2.

If we suppose, as before, that the tracer is introduced at $t = 0$ as a single administration of x_0 atoms, (5.5) can be integrated to give

$$x_1 = x_0 e^{-(K_1 + \lambda)t}$$

substituting in (5.6) we get

$$\frac{dx_2}{dt} + (\lambda + K_2)x = K_1 x_0 e^{-(K_1 + \lambda)t}$$

the solution of which is

$$\frac{x_2}{x_0} = \frac{K_1}{K_2 - K_1} e^{-\lambda t}(e^{-K_1 t} - e^{-K_2 t}) \tag{5.7}$$

For small t, this simplifies to

$$\frac{x_2}{x_0} = K_1(1 - \lambda t)t,$$

that is, an initially linear rise of activity in compartment 2 with time.

It can further be shown that x_2 rises to a maximum, at a value of t given by

$$t = \frac{1}{K_1 - K_2} \ln \frac{\lambda + K_1}{\lambda + K_2} , \tag{5.8}$$

decreasing thereafter. We can gain additional insight into the system by writing, from (5.6)

$$\ddot{x}_2 + (\lambda + K_2)\dot{x}_2 = K_1 \dot{x}_1 \tag{5.9}$$

Now, from (5.5), $\dot{x}_1 = -(K_1 + \lambda)x_1$,

that is $K_1 \dot{x}_1 = -(K_1 + \lambda)[\dot{x}_2 + (K_2 + \lambda)x_2]$ \tag{5.10}

Hence from (5.9)

$$\ddot{x}_2 + (K_1 + K_2 + 2\lambda)\dot{x}_2 + (K_1 + \lambda)(K_2 + \lambda)x_2 = 0 \tag{5.11}$$

This is the equation for the natural motion of a damped harmonic oscillator $a\ddot{x} + b\dot{x} + c = 0$. By considering the condition for heavy damping, $b^2 - 4ac > 0$, and replacing a, b, and c by the corresponding coefficients from (5.11), it is easy to show that this condition reduces to

$$(K_1 - K_2)^2 > 0 \tag{5.12}$$

which is always the case, irrespective of the relative magnitudes of K_1 and K_2, proving that a physically achievable system of this kind can nerver be inherently oscillatory in nature.

An example of the two-compartment open system is to be found in the behaviour of the thyroid gland in converting plasma iodide into thyroid hormone. If we assume that the thyroid removes iodide from the plasma at a certain rate (which in the normal subject is in the region of 1% min^{-1}), x_1 represents plasma iodide, K_1 is the rate constant for iodide removal, x_2 represents the amount of iodide in the thyroid which is then gradually removed from the iodide space, as conversion to organically bound iodine takes place. The model is defective in that it takes no account of back-transfer of iodide into the plasma, which occurs to some extent. Fig. 5.3 illustrates the behaviour of the model, which closely resembles the type of thyroid 'uptake' curves obtained in practice.

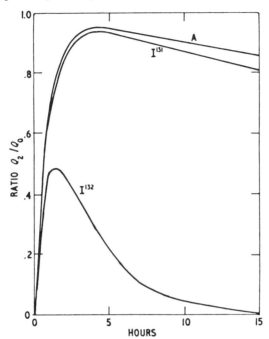

Fig. 5.3 Iodine uptake in the thyroid gland, calculated from a two-compartment model of thyroid function. Uptake curves for ^{131}I and ^{132}I are shown; curve A is corrected for radioactive decay (Spiers, 1968)

It should also be noticed that (5.7) contains λ only in the form of a multiplying factor $e^{-\lambda t}$. If all measurements are corrected for radioactive decay, the shape of the uptake curve is independent of the decay constant of the radioisotope used, and x_2/x_0 can be obtained correctly as a function of time.

A somewhat different type of 2-compartment system is shown in Fig. 5.4a, where, instead of compartment 2 being open, we assume that back-transference of the electrolyte takes place from compartment 2 to compartment 1.

Leaving out the terms relating to radioactive decay, we may write

$$\frac{dx_1}{dt} = -x_1 K_{12} + x_2 K_{21}$$

$$\frac{dx_2}{dt} = +x_1 K_{12} - x_2 K_{21}$$

(5.13)

If we assume a single input of x_0 atoms into compartment 1 at $t = 0$, this may be solved to give

$$x_1 = \frac{K_{12}}{K_{12} + K_{21}} x_0 \left[\frac{K_{21}}{K_{12}} + e^{-(K_{12} + K_{21})t} \right] \qquad (5.14a)$$

and

$$x_2 = \frac{K_{12}}{K_{12} + K_{21}} x_0 \left[1 - e^{-(K_{12} + K_{21})t} \right] \qquad (5.14b)$$

The total activity of course remains constant, and at equilibrium (that is, as $t \to \infty$)

$$\frac{x_1}{x_2} \to \frac{K_{21}}{K_{12}} \qquad (5.15)$$

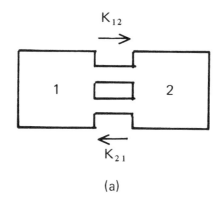

(a)

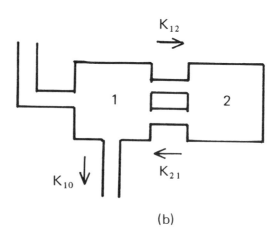

(b)

Fig. 5.4 (a) Two-compartment closed system with back-transference.
(b) Two-compartment mamillary system

This analysis can be applied to the exchange of potassium tracer atoms across the cell walls in a system consisting of plasma (compartment 1) and red cells (compartment 2) *in vitro*. Let the volume of the plasma be V, and that of a single red cell v. The number of tracer atoms entering a single red cell in time dt will be proportional to the concentration x_1/V of tracer atoms in compartment 1, the constant of proportionality being a 'fundamental' rate constant k_{12}.

Hence, for a system containing n red cells, in a time dt,

$$dx_1 = \frac{x_1}{V} n k_{12} dt \tag{5.16}$$

For back-transfer from a **single** red cell, the number of atoms dx_2 transferred in time $dt = \frac{x_2}{nv} k_{21} dt$

and from n cells, $dx_2 = \frac{x_2}{v} k_{21} dt$

Hence, at equilibrium, when $\dfrac{dx_1}{dt} = \dfrac{dx_2}{dt}$

$$\frac{x_1}{V} n k_{12} = \frac{x_2}{v} k_{21}$$

that is the ratio of **concentrations**

$$\frac{x_1}{V} \div \frac{x_2}{nv} = \frac{k_{21}}{k_{12}} \tag{5.17}$$

This ratio is the ratio of **extracellular** to **intracellular** potassium concentrations, expressed as mass per unit volume of plasma and intracellular fluid respectively, which in man is in the region of $1:40$.

As a final example we take the system illustrated in Fig. 5.4b. This is sometimes known as a two-compartment 'mamillary' system (this term denoting systems in which one or more compartments are supplied by a central compartment, as distinct from the 'catenary' nature of other systems consisting of several compartments in series), and the equations describing its behaviour may be written

$$\frac{dx_1}{dt} = -K_{10} x_1 - K_{12} x_1 + K_{21} x_2$$

$$\frac{dx_2}{dt} = +K_{12} x_1 - K_{21} x_2$$

These may be solved to give

$$x_1 = x_0(b_2 - b_1)^{-1}[(K_{21} - b_1)e^{-b_1 t} - (K_{21} - b_2)e^{-b_2 t}], \quad (5.18a)$$

and

$$x_2 = x_0(b_2 - b_1)^{-1}K_{12}[e^{-b_1 t} - e^{-b_2 t}] \quad\quad\quad (5.18b)$$

where b_1 and b_2 are the solutions of the equations

$$b_1 b_2 = K_{10} K_{21} \quad \text{and} \quad b_1 + b_2 = K_{10} + K_{21} + K_{12}.$$

Fig. 5.5 illustrates the variation of x_1 and x_2 with time. x_1 decreases rapidly at first, and more slowly thereafter. x_2 rises to a maximum and then declines towards zero.

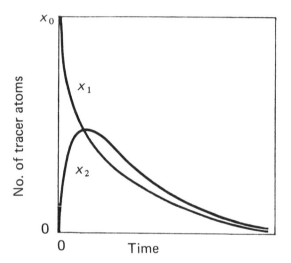

Fig. 5.5　Time-variation of the number of tracer atoms in a two-compartment mamillary system, tracer having been introduced into compartment 1 at $t = 0$
(Atkins, 1969)

The observed behaviour of isotopes of calcium and sodium (section 5.5) follows this pattern, in which an exchangeable pool (1) communicates with a 'non-exchangeable pool' (2) in the skeleton, with very small rate constants K_{12} and K_{21}.

Sufficient has been said to illustrate the general principles on which compartment theory is based. In the next section we review the general manner in which certain elements behave in the body. Much of the available knowledge in this field has been obtained by the use of radioisotopes, coupled with interpretations based on compartmental analysis along the lines just described. Diagnostic tests have arisen out of such studies. Furthermore, on the basis of such work, the potential hazards of ingestion of radioactive materials can be assessed; measurements of the body burden of radioisotopes are carried out as part of the radiological protection of occupationally-exposed workers, and have been extended to members of the public when this is deemed necessary or desirable.

5.4 TOTAL BODY WATER AND ITS SUBDIVISIONS

We have noted that water in the body behaves as a single compartment so far as a molecule of water is concerned — a molecule labelled with deuterium or tritium can diffuse freely throughout the whole of the water in the body. Equilibration requires about three hours, and if a sample of plasma is then taken the isotope dilution method may be used to determine the total body water. This method appears to be the method of choice for determining this quantity. The use of deuterium, as heavy water, has the advantage of administering no radiation dose to the patient, but this advantage is not great, because the dose involved by using tritium is only a few millirads, and is insufficient to outweigh the difficulties and expense of using deuterium.

The method appears to have a high degree of accuracy, although results obtained in animal experiments produce results 1 or 2% higher than the volumes measured directly by subsequent desiccation of the tissues. This is attributed to a small degree of exchange between tritium in water and the labile hydrogen (for example in the carboxyl groups) in fatty acids. In man the total volume of water (in the average adult male) is about 45 litres.

The water in the body may be subdivided into extracellular fluid and intracellular fluid, to which may be added transcellular fluid, to which reference has already been made. The extracellular fluid includes the plasma, and water in the gut, and may be measured directly by isotope dilution methods using suitable tracers. The sodium ion has been used for this purpose, but its value is undermined by the fact that some sodium enters the intracellular fluid and also the exchangeable part of sodium in bone. A better choice is Cl^-, although, again, there is some movement into the cells. There is also the difficulty that the radioisotopes of chlorine are inconvenient to use, ^{38}Cl with a half-life of 37 minutes only, and ^{36}Cl, with a half-life of 3×10^5 years which is difficult and expensive to produce.

However, radioactive bromine, as Br^-, has been found suitable for the determination of extracellular fluid volume. It is necessary to correct for some movement into the red cells, but the effect of this is small. Values for extracellular fluid volume in the adult male are approximately 20 litres.

The intracellular fluid volume may then be found by subtraction to be about 25 litres.

The concentration of electrolytes varies strongly in these two broadly-classified fluid compartments. For example, the exchangeable part of sodium is confined mainly to the extracellular fluid, where as potassium is found mainly in the intracellular fluid. In the next section we look at the behaviour of some important electrolytes in the body, noting particularly their distribution in various body compartments.

5.5 BEHAVIOUR OF CERTAIN ELEMENTS IN THE BODY

5.5.1 Sodium

Sodium is present in the body to the extent of about 100 g. About 60% is in the extracellular fluid, and it follows that if a radioisotope of sodium is administered, either intravenously or by mouth, it equilibrates in a few hours with extracellular sodium. Indeed, sodium radioisotopes have been used to determine the extracellular fluid volume.

Sodium is also present in bone, and part of this is exchangeable with sodium in the extracellular fluid. At 24 hours, the 'apparent dilution volume' is significantly greater than that of the extracellular fluid (27.8 litres as opposed to 20 litres), and a measurement of the specific activity of the sodium after dilution (that is in activity per unit mass of sodium as determined chemically) enables the **pool mass** of exchangeable sodium to be determined.

This quantity is less than the total amount of sodium known to be present, the balance being in a non-exchangeable compartment of bone. We can therefore begin to set up a compartment model for sodium in the body (Fig. 5.6) and the predicted behaviour of such a model bears a useful relationship to what is found in practical observations, although the extracellular compartment itself consists of several subdivisions, such as plasma, interstitial fluid, with smaller amounts in other sub-compartments. When these and other factors are taken into consideration, a more detailed model can be set up, as shown for example by Edelman and Liebman (1959).

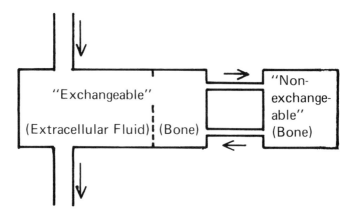

Fig. 5.6 Simplified compartment model of sodium in the body

The isotope most extensively used for short-term observations of exchangeable sodium is ^{24}Na (half-life 15 h), and excretion follows an experimental law corresponding to a biological half-life of approximately 12 days. If the longer-lived isotope ^{22}Na is used (half-life 2.6 y), retention of very small amounts is observed, evidently due to entry of a small fraction into the 'non-exchangeable' compartment, probably identifiable as mineralised bone. Burch (1962) has reported measurements of this retention, using a whole-body counter.

After administering $50\,\mu$Ci of ^{22}Na, retention of 55 nCi after 0.7 years, 31 nCi after 1.3 years, and 5 nCi after 6 years were recorded. These data do not correspond to an exponential law, the rate of decline being in fact much less rapid at the longer times. In circumstances such as this, it is sometimes possible to fit the data to a power law of the form $x = x_0 t^{-b}$. The basic premises of compartment theory break down here. Very many compartments must be involved, communicating with the extracellular fluid with different rate constants, or a continuum of rate constants. Equilibration times may be long; indeed, equilibration may never be reached.

When the above data on sodium retention are corrected for radioactive decay, it appears that an amount of tracer in the region of 1% enters the non-exchangeable pool during the time the sodium is initially in the extracellular compartment. Clearly the effective rate constants for communication with the non-exchangeable pool, and for back-transfer from it, are both very small.

5.5.2 Potassium

In contrast to sodium, potassium is present mainly in the intracellular fluid, where its concentration exceeds that in the extracellular fluid by a factor of about 40. If a potassium radioisotope such as ^{42}K or ^{43}K be introduced into the blood, it will equilibrate with all the exchangeable potassium, but on a rather longer time scale than in the case of sodium. After 24 hours, equilibration is substantially complete, with the great majority of the potassium atoms now having entered the cells, and so the total amount of exchangeable potassium in the body can be determined by measuring the amount of potassium in any sample of body fluid (say a 'spot' urine sample) and multiplying by the ratio of the activities of potassium in the body to the activity in the urine sample (or the ratio of counting rates proportional to these activities).

5.5.3 Calcium and Strontium

These elements have chemical similarities and are conveniently taken together.

The human subject contains about 1 kilogram of calcium, about 99.5% of which is in the skeleton. The remainder (about 5 g) forms an exchangeable pool which consists of the plasma, the remainder of the extracellular fluid, and the bone surfaces. Calcium introduced intravenously or orally equilibrates through the exchangeable pool within about 24 hours. A very small amount (about 0.5 g day^{-1}) exchanges with the 'non-exchangeable' calcium in bone, but, as in the case of sodium, the bone cannot be regarded as a compartment in the ordinary sense of the word. This is partly because the sites from which resorption into the plasma takes place may be different from the sites where calcium is laid down; and it is chiefly for this reason that any radioactive calcium metabolised into bone may stay there for a very long period.

The distribution of calcium in (and the exchange between) these compartments has been summarised by Dolphin and Eve (1963), and is illustrated in Fig. 5.7a.

The total transfer rate of calcium from the exchangeable pool to gut, sweat, bone and urine amounts to 0.19 per day, corresponding to a biological half-life (in the exchangeable pool) of ln2/0.19, or 3.7 days.

The behaviour of calcium in the body is important for radiological reasons, because its chemical homologue, strontium, is formed with high yield in nuclear fission in the form of ^{90}Sr, the long half-life (28 y) of which renders it potentially hazardous if ingested. Normally strontium occurs only as a trace element in the body, but a compartment model can be set up which is qualitatively similar to calcium (Fig. 5.7b). This is essentially the same compartment model as for calcium, but the rate constants are rather different. The fractional transfer rate from gut to plasma is only about half that for calcium and the fractional rate of incorporation into non-exchangeable bone is similarly less. This means that the extent to which ^{90}Sr is incorporated from the diet into bone is less than for calcium by a factor of 4; that is the 'specific activity' of ^{90}Sr (per unit mass of **calcium**) is about four times less in newly-mineralized bone than in the diet entering the gut. The hazard of ^{90}Sr is non-the-less substantial. For example, the limit of ^{90}Sr concentration in the public water supply set by current criteria of safety is as little as 4 pCi $(cm)^{-3}$.

5.5.4 Iron

This is an important element in body metabolism. It is a constituent of the haemoglobin in red blood cells (erythrocytes) upon which the oxygen transport system of the body depends. Iron is absorbed from the diet and is transported to the bone marrow, where the red blood cells are manufactured. These cells have a life of about 120 days in the blood, and when red cell destruction takes place the iron becomes reavailable for further red cell synthesis. A relatively small fraction of the dietary intake is therefore used for red cell production.

The study of iron kinetics in the body has been facilitated by radioisotopic tracer techniques using ^{59}Fe (half-life 45 days). The measurement of iron absorption from dietary intake in normal and pathological states, for example, can be carried out by tracer methods. The study of clearance rate from the plasma, and iron turnover, and the measurement of the life-time of red cells, has been made possible by tracer techniques.

Iron metabolism affords an example of the use of a 'double isotope' technique, where two different radioisotopes of the same element are used simultaneously in an investigation. If ^{59}Fe is introduced intravenously, and ^{55}Fe administered by mouth the incorporation of both into the red cells can be observed. The relative absorption (measured as percentage utilisation) of iron from the gut and from the plasma can be measured, which gives information on the uptake of iron from the dietary intake. ^{59}Fe decays by β^- decay and γ-emission, whereas ^{55}Fe is an isotope decaying by 100% orbital electron capture, emitting the characteristic x-rays of the $(Z-1)$ element, which is manganese. The two isotopes are thus readily distinguishable by the use of suitable radiation detectors.

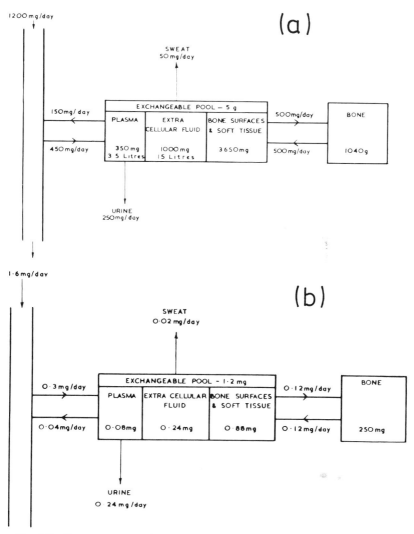

Fig. 5.7   Compartment models of (a) Calcium and (b) Strontium in the body
(Dolphin and Eve, 1963)

5.5.5 Iodine

The importance of iodine lies in the fact that it is required for the synthesis of thyroxine, a process which is carried out by the thyroid gland. Iodine is absorbed from the diet and appears in the plasmas as inorganic iodide. It is 'cleared' from the plasma by the thyroid, and in normal subjects the amount removed per minute is equivalent to the iodide content of about 25 ml of plasma, or about 0.1 μg. The iodide lost from the plasma is replaced by iodide from the iodide pool, which consists of an amount of the order of 100 μg, situated mainly in the extracellular fluid. (The body contains 10-15 mg of iodine, mainly organically bound, of which the great majority is located in the thyroid gland.)

The function of the thyroid can be analysed into 3 stages: (a) the uptake of iodide from plasma (b) the conversion of iodide into thyroxine and (c) the secretion of thyroxine into the blood. Radioisotopes can measure the rate constant for the first and last of these processes.

The percentage of administered iodine taken up by the thyroid is shown in Fig. 5.8, which is a distribution curve obtained from data relating to 400 patients who were judged, by other criteria, to be normal in respect of thyroid function. The spread is rather wide, but the curve has a well-defined maximum, which is in the region of 30%.

The significance of the thyroid uptake test lies in the fact that in abnormal states of the gland the percentage uptake may be substantially different from this value. For thyrotoxic (hyperactive) glands, the range given is 45-95% after 24 hours (median about 70%) and for myxoedematous patients (underactive thyroid) the figure will be 20% or less. This therefore forms a diagnostic test which has been applied very widely indeed over the last 30 years, although it should be added that its use is declining in the face of more modern methods based on the determination of iodide and organic (protein-bound) iodine in the blood, and also direct measurement of thyroxine levels in plasma at appropriate times after administration.

To carry out the thyroid uptake test, a few microcuries of ^{131}I are administered orally, and a scintillation counter is positioned against the neck in order to record the counting rate as a function of time. If several measurements are made following the administration of the tracer, the geometry must be accurately reproducible. The system is calibrated against standards, and is collimated so as to reduce as far as possible the interfering effect of plasma iodine. A correction for this can be applied by measuring the counting rate when the counter is placed against some other part of the body, for example the thigh. Normally measurements at one or two times only (for example 6 hours and 24 hours) are needed.

In the thyrotoxic patient, the iodide is cleared from the blood more rapidly than in normal subjects, and the condition is characterised also by the rapid re-appearance, in the plasma, of iodine in the form of thyroxine bound to protein molecules.

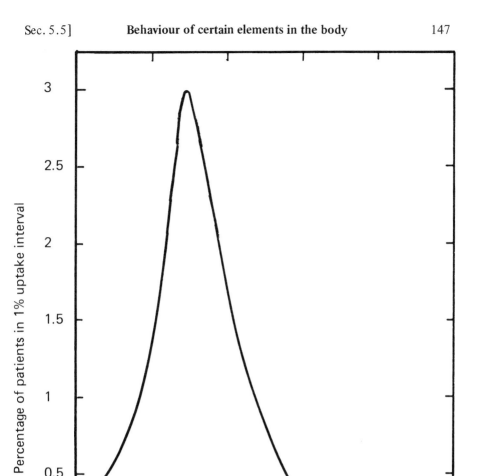

Fig. 5.8 The frequency distribution of thyroid uptake in normal subjects
(Silver, 1962)

The radiation dose delivered to the thyroid in this test is in the range 1–10 rad, which is now generally considered to be somewhat high. The radiation dose can be substantially reduced, by the use of ^{132}I, and values only about 100 mrad are quoted when this radioisotope is used. ^{132}I is a β and γ emitter with a half-life of 2.3 hours. It is obtained from a ^{132}Te generator. ^{132}Te decays by β-decay to ^{132}I, so that the latter isotope can be 'milked' from the ^{132}Te periodically. If ^{132}I is used, the thyroid counting rate must be measured at an earlier time (see Fig. 5.3), for example 2 or 4 hours rather than 6 hours or more. This still allows the thyroid trapping function to be measured, but precludes observation of the 'organification' of iodine and its subsequent transport out of the thyroid.

The use of the shorter-lived isotope means that greater activities can be used, thereby obtaining better counting statistics, whilst still maintaining the absorbed radiation dose at a low level.

^{131}I is produced in nuclear fission, and because of its volatility when in elemental form (I_2) it is recognised to be a potential environmental hazard, in the event of an accidental release of radioactivity from a nuclear reactor or nuclear processing plant. It can in principle be absorbed by man directly from the atmosphere, or can be ingested by cattle, in which case it appears subsequently in milk and hence enters the human food-chain. Iodine metabolism has therefore been studied intensively for reasons which are additional to its importance in clinical medicine.

5.6 SCANNING AND IMAGING TECHNIQUES

We have seen how various radioisotopes follow an established route within the body and are known to exhibit a differential of concentration in different parts of the body. It follows that much information can, in principle, be obtained by using external radiation detectors to monitor the movement of radioisotopes and to measure the activity within an organ, either to compare it with the activity of surrounding tissues or to study the distribution within the organ itself. Such measurements are possible if the radioisotope is a γ-emitter, so that the emitted radiation can in fact emerge from a relatively deep-seated organ, and be detected by instruments placed on or near the body surface.

The simplest external radiation detector consists of a scintillation counter placed close to the region under investigation and connected to its associated electronics, which will normally include a single-channel pulse-height analyser. Such a detector will normally be shielded against unwanted radiation, for example background radiation, or radiation from other parts of the body. It will also be fitted with a collimator to limit the area to which the counter is sensitive. If it is desired to look at an area several centimetres across, the wide-angle collimator in Fig. 5.9a may be satisfactory. The narrow-angle collimator in Fig 5.9b would be suitable for smaller areas. However, if it is desired to measure the activity along a line, or over a 2-dimensional area, the resolution of the system will be an important parameter, and will need to be sufficiently good to delineate with adequate accuracy the organ being investigated. The focussing type of collimator shown in Fig. 5.9c is used extensively when good resolution is desired, as in the moving detector rectilinear scanner, and can achieve a substantial improvement in sensitivity over the narrow angle collimator. It will be immediately apparent that the resolution will be adversely affected if the radiation is able to penetrate

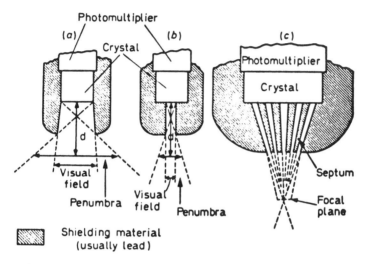

Fig. 5.9 (a) Wide-angle collimator. (b) Narrow-angle collimator. (c) Focussing collimator (Trott, 1971)

the walls ('septa') separating the collimator channels. Clearly the choice of gamma-ray energy and wall thickness are crucial design parameters, if optimum performance is to be achieved. The system will normally be required to display a region of enhanced uptake, and will operate most effectively, if the differential uptake of the administered labelled material is as large as possible. Several factors will thus operate to determine the minimum detectable size of a region of enhanced uptake, and an understanding of these factors requires detailed consideration of the quantitative behaviour of the many pharmaceutical agents which have been investigated for differential uptake. It may be said that this minimum detectable size is rarely less than 1 cm, and will often be greater than this. In the special case of thyroid imaging by meas of radioactive iodine, the differential uptake is so large that features considerably smaller than this can be detected, and a 'resolution' of 2–3 mm can be attained, enabling the point-to-point variations (which may be considerable) in uptake to be imaged in some detail.

    To obtain a two-dimensional scan, the counter is mounted on a mechanism which can move across the area undergoing investigation, together with a small stepping motion between each translation, so that the area can be covered completely. To display the information obtained, a marker can be caused to move synchronously across a recorder, printing a point after the passage of a given number of counts through the detection system. An increase in counting rate will thus be observed as an increased density of points printed on the chart. Another method makes use of a small light-source moving over a photographic film, the brightness of the source, or the frequency of its flashes, being proportional to the dector counting rate. This enables the data to be presented on transparent film which may then be viewed on a conventional viewing box, as used for diagnostic x-radiographs. Yet another method of display consists of a system of coloured inked ribbons, actuated by a ratemeter, placed between a regularly activated 'tapper' and the recording paper which moves in synchronism with the radiation detector. In this way the counting rates can be represented as a graded colour scale, and the system of colours can be chosen to confer maximum visibility on the recorded image.

An electronic recording system, involving no mechanical motion, can be used in which the impulses from the detector are transmitted to the screen of a storage oscilloscope, building up an image point-by-point as the detector executes its scan across the field undergoing investigation.

Systems using a single radiation detector suffer from the fundamental drawback that much of the available information is wasted — the device can record the activity from only one picture element at a time. Accordingly, much effort has been devoted to the development of radiation cameras, by means of which the radiation output from the whole field of view can be measured by the detector and then displayed on a storage tube. Such a system necessarily requires that the detector system shall be 'position-sensitive' and that there shall be a one-to-one correspondence between the point (in the detector assembly) at which an 'event' is detected and the point (on the display) at which the event is displayed. This is achieved by fabricating the detector crystal in the form of a circular slab (which may be $10''$–$12''$ in diameter) and arranging for it to be 'viewed' by a matrix of several photomultipliers. The amount of light reaching each photomultiplier from an 'event' will therefore depend on the coordinates of the point at which the γ-photon is absorbed. In a radiation camera this information (that is the relative signal amplitudes from the photomultipliers) is converted into x- and y-signals which are then used to activate the display. This principle is illustrated in Fig. 5.10. Up to 19 photomultipliers are used in some assemblies of this type. A gamma-camera requires the use of a 'honeycomb' type of collimator in front of the sintillator, and requires also that the patient be positioned as closely as possible to the collimator mounting.

One of the most successful areas of application of radioisotope scanning and imaging has been in the field of brain scanning. Counters placed near the head are relatively unaffected by radiation from other parts of the body; furthermore, the relatively small size of the head allows the emitted radiation to emerge with relatively little attenuation. A more fundamental reason for success lies in the particular properties of brain tissue, in that the permeability of the cell walls is particularly low when compared with other tissues. This means that radio-activity introduced intravenously enters normal cells only to a small degree, but apparently to a much greater degree in the abnormal cells found in brain tumours. The penetration of the 'blood–brain barrier' allows visualisation of tumourous tissue to a marked extent, although it should be added that this mechanism may in some circumstances be supplemented by the increased amount of extracellular fluid in some tumours, into which radioisotopes introduced into the blood may diffuse freely. Furthermore, the blood–brain barrier may be disturbed, and its permeability increased, by other factors, such as a brain injury, not associated with malignant disease. Radioisotopes used for brain-scanning include ^{131}I-labelled human serum albumin, ^{74}As as arsenate or arsenite, and ^{99m}Tc as pertechnetate. This last radioisotope decays by an isomeric transition, emitting γ-rays of 190 keV, with no β-radiation (apart from some conversion electrons). Its energy is thus ideal for imaging by the gamma-camera. Furthermore, its short half-life ($\sim$6 h) means that relatively large activities may be administered without exceed-ing a moderately low radiation dose to the patient. Other radiopharmaceuticals used for brain scanning, together with some procedural details, have been

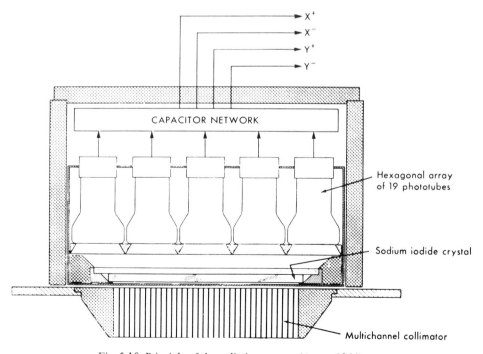

Fig. 5.10 Principle of the radiation camera (Anger, 1964)

described by Mallard (1971), who also gives an extensive bibliography relating to the very considerable research which has been carried out in this particular field of radioisotope imaging.

The selective uptake of other reagents in particular organs or glands has been exploited for imaging. For example, the pancreas, the organ in which certain digestive enzymes are produced, may be imaged by the use of selenomethionine labelled with ^{75}Se, this being the selenium analogue of methionine, an amino acid which is incorporated into newly-synthesised protein. Pancreatic function can thus be assessed by imaging techniques. A related technique is that of liver imaging, which is found to be practicable using either a scanning technique or a gamma-camera. Thyroid scanning has already been referred to, and is used as a means of delineating non-functioning thyroid tissue, or looking for residual function following thyroid ablation by isotope therapy. Functioning metastases also may be detected by their iodine uptake.

For more detailed descriptions of these important techniques, and for additional applications, the reader is referred to the accounts given by Trott (1971) and by Mallard (1971), and the detailed descriptions by Wagner (1968).

5.7 THERAPY WITH RADIOACTIVE ISOTOPES

Our discussion so far has been concerned largely with the study of physiological function, and it is essential that the radiation dose to any part of the body be insufficient to cause any modification of function. However, if substantially higher activities are administered, the possibility of modifying the function becomes real, opening the way to therapeutic uses of internally administered radioisotopes.

This was recognised at an early stage in the use of radioiodine for thyroid studies, when it became apparent that an overactive thyroid can be controlled by the administration of a therapeutic amount of ^{131}I as iodide. To achieve effective control in cases of thyrotoxicosis, radiation doses in the region of 7500 rads to the thyroid are required. To obtain irradiation at this level, administered activities of several millicuries of ^{131}I are needed, that is about 1000 times larger than would be used for diagnostic work. This treatment for thryotoxicosis has been highly successful, and in 1962 Silver was able to write that over 100,000 patients had been treated for this condition since 1948. The radiation dosimetry for this type of treatment is complex. Previously obtained data on thyroid uptake in the same patient would not necessarily apply when the gland is in the course of change, due to radiobiological damage; non-uniformity in the uptake of iodine means that the absorbed radiation dose will be non-uniform, precluding accurate assessment of dose; furthermore, the radiation dose to other tissues may become clinically significant, as for example the dose to the erythropoietic (red blood-cell forming) tissue in the bone marrow, giving rise to clinical side effects which should naturally be avoided if possible.

Radioiodine therapy has been extended to the treatment of thyroid carcinoma. In such a situation one is aiming at the destruction of all thyroid tissue, and for this purpose a radiation dose of up to 30,000 rads may be needed, necessitating the administration of up to 100 mCi of ^{131}I. The amount which may be administered is limited by radiation effects on other tissues, notably the bone-marrow, as discussed above.

One further point should be made regarding the therapeutic use of iodine for thyroid cancer. If there are metastases, they may be capable of some degree of function, in the sense of taking up iodide and at least commencing the process of synthesis into thyroxine or its precursors. Radioiodine is thus, in principle able to deliver a radiation dose to metastases wherever they occur, even if they have not been located or identified. This is an important feature of the treatment.

Another successful field of radioisotope therapy has been the use of ^{32}P for treatment of the bone-marrow disease **polycythaemia vera**. This condition is characterised by excessive activity of the blood-forming tissues in the marrow. The chemical and radioactive characteristics of ^{32}P (β-emitter; no γ radiation except Bremsstrahlung; half-life 14.3 days) make it very suitable for the treatment of this disease. Activities of a few millicuries are administered intravenously, and about 40% of the administered activity normally reaches the erythropoietic tissue. The main difficulty in this form of treatment lies in the amount of total-body radiation to which the patient is exposed, due to the circulating ^{32}P. The total-body radiation dose from the β-particles is increased by the Bremsstrahlung produced as a consequence of the somewhat high β-particle energy. The amount of total-body radiation normally sets a limit to the amount of activity which may be safely administered.

Radioisotopes in colloidal form are used for the treatment of certain neoplastic conditions of the membrane surrounding the pleural cavity, which is the space in the thorax between the chest wall and the lung. The production of fluid by these linings is clinically undesirable, and these 'pleural effusions' can be controlled by the injection of colloidal gold (as ^{198}Au) or ^{32}P-labelled colloidal chromium phosphate. The same technique has been used for the treatment of neoplasms in lymph nodes.

5.8 GASEOUS RADIOISOTOPES

5.8.1 Introduction

A development of particular interest has been the study of radioactive isotopes in gaseous form. As might be expected, these lend themselves particularly to the study of lung function, and of the gas exchange processes which occur between gases in the lung, and the blood supply with which the lung is perfused. Radioactive gases are of value both for elucidating some fundamental aspects of gas exchange and also for divising diagnostic tests for use in cases of suspected disorders in lung function.

Gases used for this work may conveniently be divided into two classes – first, certain noble gases, particularly radioisotopes of xenon and krypton, may be prepared in a form suitable for clinical administration either by inhalation or intravenous injection, for the investigations of ventilation (the amount of air inspired during normal breathing) and perfusion (the rate at which blood passes through the lungs). The other class consists of radioisotopes of certain light elements, notably oxygen (^{15}O), nitrogen (^{13}N) and carbon (^{11}C). These have several features which commend them for this type of work – they are constituents of air, and therefore follow the normal physiological processes of respiration. Further, they are short-lived (with half-lives of 2 m, 10 m, and 20 m respectively), with obvious advantages, so far as minimising radiation doses is concerned. And thirdly, they are all positron emitters, so that there is always some accompanying annihilation radiation, which facilitates external detection by scintillation counters placed over the chest wall. In the case of ^{11}C, its value relies on the ability to convert the element into suitable gaseous compounds, notably $^{11}CO_2$ and ^{11}CO.

5.8.2 Preparation

The isotope of xenon most often encountered in this type of work is ^{133}Xe, which decays by β^--emission (half-life 5.3 days) to stable ^{133}Cs, emitting a gamma-ray at 81 keV. ^{133}Xe is produced by neutron capture in ^{132}Xe (natural abundance 27%) and is also a product of uranium fission. It is therefore readily prepared by reactor irradiation, or by extraction from irradiated fuel elements. It can be made available in gaseous form, or in a solution of isotonic saline for intravenous use.

The short-lived isotopes of the light elements listed above are prepared by charged-particle bombardment in a cyclotron, the most favoured reactions being

$$^{14}N(d,n)^{15}O$$

$$^{12}C(d,n)^{13}N$$

and $^{10}B(d,n)^{11}C$ or $^{11}B(d,2n)^{11}C$.

In order to produce samples of ^{15}O in elementary form, deuterons of 3–6 MeV enter a bombardment chamber through a thin aluminium window. Nitrogen gas (with about 4% oxygen carrier) flows through the chamber under slight pressure, and then on to the processing and purifying system. It is passed over soda-lime to remove oxides of nitrogen, and then over activated charcoal to remove other impurities, such as traces of ozone. ^{15}O can be produced at an activity of the order of 200 mCi ℓ^{-1} and is available for dilution with air for clinical administration. ^{15}O-labelled carbon dioxide may be made by passing the labelled oxygen over charcoal heated to $500°C$. The equilibrium reaction

$$3O_2 + 4C \rightleftharpoons 2CO + 2CO_2$$

is established, and if the product is then passed over copper at $850°C$, the CO is oxidised to CO_2. To produce ^{15}O-labelled carbon monoxide the charcoal reaction is carried out at $850°C$, when the equilibrium favours the production of CO, the CO_2 being then removable by passing over soda-lime.

The production of ^{13}N may be achieved by bombarding a graphite target using a suitable sweep gas, or by using CO_2 as the combined target material and sweep gas. The ^{13}N may be diluted to a few mCi ℓ^{-1} for breathing, or alternatively solutions in isotonic saline may be prepared.

The preparation of ^{11}C calls for the bombardment of boron. This is most conveniently carried out by using boric oxide B_2O_3, which may be allowed to melt during bombardment in order to assist in the evolution of the gaseous products. Argon may be used as sweep gas, with CO or CO_2 carrier, as appropriate. Chemical processing, using principles similar to those outlined above, ensures that the labelled product is radiochemically pure. If the product is required in carrier-free form, a sweep gas of hydrogen ensures that the product gases will be reduced to ^{11}CO, without the need to introduce carbon monoxide as carrier. If helium is used, the ^{11}C activity appears mainly as $^{11}CO_2$.

As a further example of a gaseous isotope in clinical use, the short-lived krypton isotope ^{81m}Kr (half-life 13 s) may be cited. This is prepared by cyclotron bombardment of sodium bromide to form ^{81}Rb by the $^{79}Br(\alpha, 2n)^{81}Rb$ and similar reactions. The ^{81}Rb is prepared on a column and generates equilibrium activities of ^{81m}Kr which may be eluted and made available for use as required. The rubidium parent decays with a half-life of 4.7 hours, which is not too short to prevent its use on an increasing scale at centres which are not too remote from cyclotron facilities.

5.8.3 Physiological principles and clinical applications

The ability of the lungs, or a specified region of a lung, to take in air during inspiration is termed ventilation, or regional ventilation. In deep breathing the ventilation is of course increased, and the relative ventilation of different regions of the lung changes, parts near the apices of the lungs which are relatively poorly ventilated during quiet breathing becoming more ventilated in deep breathing. Another important parameter is the blood flow, which is the volume of blood passing through the lungs per unit time. This definition may similarly be extended to discrete regions of the lung, if the region can be defined precisely.

We need to consider the differing solubilities of gases in water or plasma. In the case of gases which are only sparingly soluble, the quantity dissolving is proportional to the partial pressure of the gas in the gaseous phase, which implies that the volume dissolving per unit volume of liquid is independent of partial pressure, if the volume is measured at that pressure. If n_{soln} and n_{gas} are the number of molecules of gas per unit volume of solution and gas respectively, we may write (Fig. 5.11a)

$$\frac{n_{soln}}{n_{gas}} = \alpha, \tag{5.19}$$

This constancy of α is an expression of **Henry's law** for the solution of gases in liquids, **and is true for the minute partial pressures associated with radioactive atoms or molecules.**

α depends strongly upon temperatue, falling as the temperature rises. For nitrogen at body temperature $\alpha = 0.012$ for solution in plasma (slightly less than

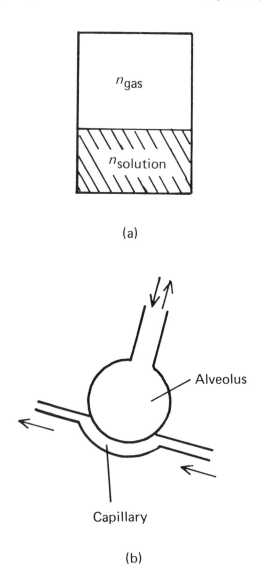

(a)

(b)

Fig. 5.11 (a,b) Illustrating gas-exchange in the lung

in water because of the presence of dissolved salts in the plasma), and for argon $\alpha = 0.026$. Carbon dioxide is an example of a more soluble gas, for which α (plasma; $37°C$) $= 0.54$. If chemical combination occurs, the situation is more complex. For oxygen, $\alpha = 0.023$, but its behaviour in whole blood is conditioned by the fact that it combines chemically with haemoglobin in the red cells to form oxyhaemoglobin, this being the mechanism by which oxygen is transported to the body tissues. The relation between the partial pressure and the amount of oxygen in solution is not linear, and requires the setting up of the 'dissociation curve' for oxygen in blood.

For xenon, $\alpha = 0.10$ in water, but is 0.18 in blood, because of some attachment to the haemoglobin. Xenon is therefore a gas of intermediate solubility. Krypton is somewhat less soluble than xenon, though considerably more so than nitrogen or argon.

Air enters the lungs through the main bronchi, and is then distributed to successively smaller airways known successively as bronchioles, respiratory bronchioles, and alveolar ducts. These in turn lead to a complex of minute sacs, or alveoli, which are the ultimate destination of inspired air. Venous blood is supplied to the lungs via the pulmonary artery which, by successive branchings, leads to very many capillaries separated from the alveoli by membranes. It is across these membranes that gas exchange occurs — oxygen entering the blood from the alveoli, and carbon dioxide crossing in the opposite direction simultaneously. The sites of gas exchange may be represented schematically as in Fig. 5.11b. Interpretation of the observations following inspiration or intravenous injection of radioactive gases therefore depends ultimately on a knowledge of the physical processes of gas exchange occurring at these locations.

Reverting to the context of radioactive gases, the simplest type of measurement is that in which a labelled gas (for example air labelled with oxygen-15) is inhaled during a single deep breath, the subject then holding his breath for, say, 15 or 20 seconds. If external counters are placed close to the chest wall (for example 2 counters, one over each lung) they will record a rapid rise during inspiration, and a slow decline during breath-holding. A rather more rapid decline will then take place when normal breathing is resumed, as the residual active gas is 'washed-out' by the normal breathing process.

In the normal subject the tracings obtained from each lung will be essentially similar and any deficiency of either ventilation or blood flow in one lung relative to the other will be revealed by comparing the two traces. The normal decline of oxygen-15 activity during breath holding is found to be approximately linear, as oxygen is steadily taken up by the blood. This has been found to be at a rate which is low near the apices, becoming progressively greater near the base of the lung, and is in the region of 1–2% per second, although it should be noted that the rate of disappearance of (stable) oxygen from the lungs is in fact less than this due to considerable back-diffusion of oxygen from venous blood back into the alveoli.

Tracings comparing upper and lower regions of the lung are shown in Fig. 5.12, where a single inspiration of ^{15}O-labelled air followed by breath holding is illustrated. The ventilation and 'clearance rates' are both less in the apical regions (even allowing for the reduced thickness of lung near the apex in the case of ventilation) but both these quantities become more equal during exercise.

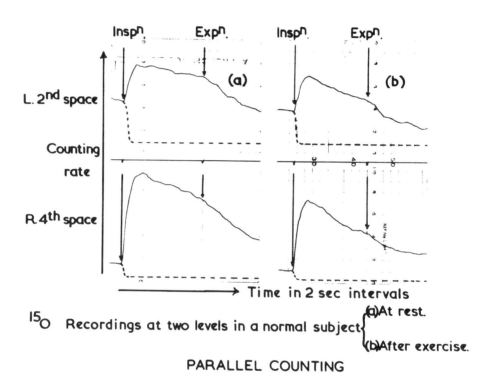

Fig. 5.12 'Clearance' of ^{15}O-labelled air at two levels of the lung. (a) resting (b) on exercise (Dollery *et al.*, 1960)

Lung function studies are normally designed with reference to the solubility of the radioactive gas; if a soluble gas is needed (for example for comparison of clearance rates from different regions of a lung or comparison between the two lungs), ^{15}O-labelled carbon dioxide, which is cleared very rapidly from the lungs, may be used. A pair of tracings obtained with ^{15}O-labelled carbon dioxide is illustrated in Fig. 5.13.

If a sparingly-soluble gas is required, ^{13}N-labelled nitrogen or ^{133}Xe are usually preferred. As an example of the use of a sparingly-soluble gas, let us consider the information obtainable from the inspiration of ^{13}N-labelled nitrogen in a single breath. The initial counter readings will be proportional to regional ventilation, but unless the measurements are confined to two counters, left and right, at the same level and in a normal subject, the constant of proportionality in the readings from each counter will in general be different, because of the varying thicknesses of lung being viewed at different positions over the thorax. If however the subject now breathes steadily in a closed circuit system the activity will equilibrate throughout the system, and the **ratio of counting-rate during breath-holding to that after equilibration** will be proportional to **the regional ventilation per unit alveolar volume**, and the constant of proportionality will be truly constant for a given procedure and a given counting system. The results from all parts of the lungs may thereafter be compared directly. The use of a poorly-soluble gas in this way is the basis of a clinically useful test.

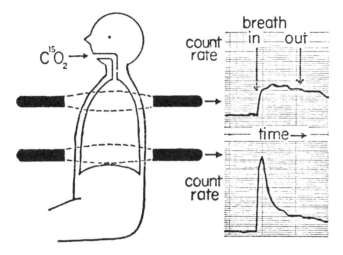

Fig. 5.13 Relative measurements of regional blood flow using ^{15}O-labelled carbon dioxide (West, 1963)

On the other hand, if the labelled nitrogen be dissolved in isotonic saline and injected into a vein, the initial reading will depend on **regional blood flow**. Because the gas is poorly soluble, it will pass almost entirely into the alveolae during the first passage through the lung. If the patient again breaths steadily into a closed system, the ration of 'initial' to 'equilibrium' counting rates will now given the **regional blood-flow per unit alveolar volume**.

The use of xenon–133, or, where available, nitrogen–13 thus lends itself to the investigation of lung function in normal and pathological states. Yet other possibilities have further extended the value of this technique. For example, we have noted that a poorly-soluble gas introduced intravenously should move almost entirely into the alveolae during passage through the lung. If, then, activity is detected in arterial blood, it signifies the passage of blood directly from the right to the left side of the heart without passing through the lung. These right-to-left shunts represent a heart defect and may be indicative of the need for surgical intervention and repair.

5.8.4 Techniques of measurement

Radiation from inhaled radioactive gases is measured by means of scintillation counters placed close to the chest wall. We have seen that ^{15}O, ^{13}N and ^{11}C are all positron emitters. They decay to the ground state of the daughter nucleus, so that only annihilation radiation is emitted, and this is sufficiently penetrating to be detectable from all depths within the thorax. By suitable collimator design, a good degree of regional discrimination can be achieved, and it is often useful to arrange the counters in pairs, in front of and behind the chest wall, with their outputs connected to the same scaler or ratemeters, The response of such a pair of counters is illustrated in Fig. 5.14, in which lines of equal response are plotted on a contour diagram. The spatial resolution of such a system is adequate for many applications, although there is always the possibility that an area of reduced uptake would be masked by the much larger activity from surrounding regions in the same field of view. Multihole 'focussing' collimators of the kind described in section 5.6 would give an improved spatial descrimination but the difficulty in detecting regions of reduced uptake would remain.

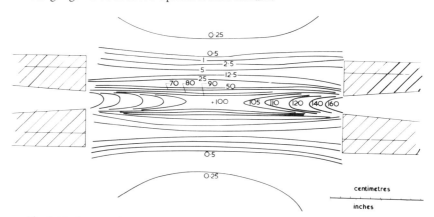

Fig. 5.14 Iso-count response curves of a pair of scintillation counters connected additively (Dyson *et al.*, 1960)

These problems may be overcome by utilising the fact that the annihilation of a positron and an electron give rise to two photons, each of energy 511 keV, travelling in opposite directions. By setting up two counters in coincidence, the response of the system can be confined strictly to the volume of space between the two detectors. By suitable choice of aperture the resolution can be made arbitrarily fine, although the progressive loss of sensitivity as the aperture is reduced sets a practical limit to this. In practice an aperture of about 4 cm is small enough to give adequate resolution. Conical collimators are not required, and the response of such a coincidence system is illustrated in Fig. 5.15.

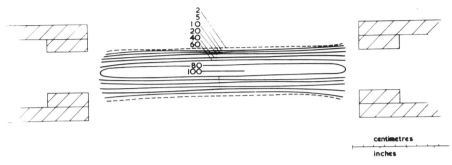

Fig. 5.15   Iso-count response curves of a pair of scintillation counters connected in coincidence with the source in air (Dyson *et al.*, 1960)

A further advantage of such a system is that if such curves are obtained with the source surrounded by a medium, the depth-response function is unaffected by this. Referring to Fig. 5.16 we see that, if the response in the absence of a medium is given by $N(x)$, the presence of a medium of linear absorption coefficient μ reduces the photons travelling in the two directions by factors of $e^{-\mu(D + x)}$ and $e^{-\mu(D - x)}$ respectively. The coincidence counting rate, which is proportional to the product of the probabilities of photons being detected in the two channels, will now be reduced by a factor of

$$e^{-\mu(D + x)} e^{-\mu(D - x)}$$
$$= e^{-2\mu D}, \tag{5.20}$$

which is independent of x. In these expressions x is the co-ordinate (abscissa) of the source position, measured from an origin mid-way between the two detectors, and D is the distance of each detector from that origin.

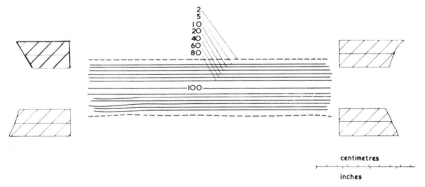

Fig. 5.16   Iso-count response curves of a pair of scintillation counters connected in coincidence, with the source in a medium (Dyson, 1960)

Concidence counting systems have been described by several authors for example Sweet *et al.* (1959), Dyson (1960) and Matthews (1964). They have been found to be of particular value in brain scanning, as well as in lung function studies, although the relatively low counting rates present a difficulty in the study of slowly-varing quantities such as clearance-rate, where the statistical fluctuations preclude accurate measurement.

The other radioisotopes mentioned so far, viz. ^{133}Xe and ^{81m}Kr, are γ-emitters. ^{133}Xe emits γ-radiation at 81 keV, and ^{81m}Kr at 190 keV. The radiation from both these isotopes are readily collimated, and are conveniently detected by scintillation counters together with conventional counting equipment.

The development of the gamma-camera has enabled short-term variations in activity to be followed in detail. By using a storage type of display, the distribution of activity can be measured during breath holding. Alternatively, kinetic studies can be carried out, following, for example, an intravenous injection of activity. The 13-second ^{81m}Kr has particular potential in this respect, as its 190 keV γ-radiation is in the range which is ideal for imaging. Some ventilation and perfusion studies using this method with ^{81m}Kr have been described by Jones *et al.* (1970) and Yano *et al.* (1970).

Other gaseous isotopes which are used in this field are ^{85m}Kr and ^{85}Kr. The last-named has a half-life of 10.8 y, but is essentially a β-emitter, as γ-rays are produced in only 0.4% of disintegrations. It is not suitable for external counting but can be assayed in blood samples or in expired air.

The metastable ^{85m}Kr (half-life 4.4 hr) has been described as being suitable for lung function studies, with γ-rays of 150 keV (74%) and 305 keV (13%), which are in the correct energy range for use with γ-cameras. The isotopes ^{79}Kr, ^{135}Xe and ^{127}Xe have also been noted as being potentially useful. The preparation of these isotopes has been described by Clark and Buckingham, to whose account the reader is referred for details.

5.8.5 Other aspects of radioactive gases

Interest in the study of radioactive gases is not confined to their uses for investigation of pulmonary or cardiac function. The natural radioactivity in the environment includes the gaseous members of the natural radioactive series, which were referred to in Chapter 4. Radium (as ^{226}Ra) is widely dispersed in the earth's crust, and because radon (^{222}Rn) is the immediate daughter product of radium, it escapes from soil and rocks to form detectable amounts in the atmosphere. It is then inhaled and decays into ^{218}Po(RaA), the so-called 'active deposit'. This, and further decay products, may remain in the body to give a contribution to the 'natural' radiation dose. Radium itself is present in the body – largely in bone – to the extent of the order of 10^{-10} Ci. Its decay to radon results in the appearance of radon in the breath, and it is known that 60–70% of radon is exhaled, the raminder being retained in the form of the active deposit. The annual radiation dose received by the body due to internal sources of ^{226}Ra is about 0.6 mrad to bone, and that due to ^{222}Rn and its short-lived decay products is of the order of 0.3 mrad. These doses appear small compared with the total of 100 mrad per annum from all natural sources, but it must be remembered that the dose from radium and its decay products is predominantly due to α-particles with a relative biological efficiency (or RBE – *q.v.* Chapter 6) which may be of the order of 10 or more. This must be used as a weighting factor when comparing the potential biological effect of α-emitters with that of the other contributing radiations.

Particular importance must be attached to the possibility of accidental ingestion of radium. The element is little-used nowadays, but was formerly used for the painting of luminous dials. This resulted in the accidental ingestion of toxic amounts of radium, and in a few cases anaemia and other conditions developed leading to death within a few years. Careful investigation of radium workers has established an abnormally high incidence of malignant disease with eventual death from this cause. The cumulative radiation dose to bone from the amounts known to have lodged there is sufficient to account for this.

During the years immediately following the discovery of radioactivity, radium salts were on occasion prescribed medicinally, and similar effects are known to have occurred in patients treated in this manner.

The production of a radioactive gas *in situ* arises in an interesting way in connection with the *in vivo* determination of calcium in the body by neutron activation analysis. The latter group of techniques, whereby an element is assayed by measuring the radioactivity induced by irradiation with neutrons, is discussed in Chapter 6, but one particular method should be referred to here. This is based on the production of the radioisotope ^{37}Ar by the reaction ^{40}Ca$(n,\alpha)^{37}$Ar. As more than 99% of total body calcium is found in the skeleton, the behaviour of the gaseous ^{37}Ar activity presents an interesting problem in radioisotope kinetics. The gas is observed to be exhaled in the breath and, in principle at least, the amount of calcium in the body can be determined by collecting the activity exhaled over a measured period and determining it by an absolute method. The variation of exhaled activity with time is however influenced by several factors, notably the rate constant for diffusion of the activity from mineral bone into the blood, from which it will then be transferred rapidly to the exhaled breath, following the principles outlined for poorly-soluble gases in section 5.8.3 above. However, trapping in, and subsequent slow diffusion from, the mineralised part of bone is a factor requiring to be taken into consideration. For example, Bigler *et al.* (1976) found that 30% of the ^{37}Ar activity remained trapped essentially permanently, probably in bone crystals. Furthermore, it is probable that some argon may dissolve in fat and fatty tissue, to be released gradually over a period of time. The study of exhalation curves obtained by this method, and also following intravenous injection of xenon as ^{133}Xe, when solubility in fat certainly plays an important role, has been reported by Leach *et al.* (1978). The behaviour of the noble gases within the body is clearly a subject of considerable fundamental interest.

5.9 INTERNAL DOSIMETRY OF RADIOISOTOPES

Some knowledge of the radiation dose absorbed from internally administered radioisotopes is often required. When devising a diagnostic test requiring the administration of radioactive materials, it is necessary to know the amount of any radiation likely to be delivered as a result of this, in order to assess the level of any radiation hazard involved. It is also important to establish that the radiation dose is insufficient to bring about any change in function in any of the systems undergoing investigation. Normally this can be ensured with a high degree of reliability. Calculations are much more difficult than the corresponding calculations for external sources of radiation, such as x-ray beams used in diagnostic radiology, and are subject to much greater uncertainty.

When using radioisotopes for therapeutic purposes it is, of course, essential to calculate as carefully as possible the dose to the tissues undergoing irradiation (that is the thyroid, or, in the case of ^{32}P treatment of polycythaemia, the erythropoietic tissue) and also to assess the dose to other organs in the body. This dose will often not be negligible when using the large amounts of activity required for therapy, and the dose likely to be sustained by, for example, the gonads will normally be calculated in the course of treatment planning. The dose to blood and erythropoietic tissue is also of some consequence in all therapeutic procedures.

Radiation doses originating from occupational or environmental hazards are frequently calculated, in order to arrive at some assessment of risk, or at least to carry out a comparison with the dose received from unavoidable natural sources, such as natural radioactivity and cosmic radiation.

The simplest case is one in which radioactivity is uniformly distributed throughout a homogeneous sphere, the radius of which is large compared with the mean free path of the radiation. Except near the surface, equilibrium conditions exist, and the amount of radiation originating in a small volume (but being absorbed elsewhere) will equal the energy deposited in the volume from surrounding regions of the sphere. This condition will be achieved in the case of a β-emitter distributed in a sphere with a radius of a few centimetres, because the mean free path of β-particles rarely exceeds a few millimetres in material of unit density. As an example, if we consider a sphere of unit density containing ^{32}P (a pure β^--emitter with $E_{max} = 1.68$ MeV) at a concentration of $1\,\mu$Ci (ml)$^{-1}$, the only additional quantity needed is the mean energy per disintegration. Let this be $\bar{E}_\beta$. Then the energy released per second per unit volume within the sphere will be given by

$$3.7 \times 10^4 \bar{E}_\beta.$$

If charged particle equilibrium exists, the dose rate may be seen to be given by

$$D_\beta = 3.7 \times 10^4 \bar{E}_\beta \, 1.6 \times 10^{-13} \times 10^5 \text{ rad sec}^{-1}$$
$$= 5.92 \bar{E}_\beta \times 10^{-4} \text{ rad sec}^{-1}, \qquad (5.21)$$

with $\bar{E}_\beta$ in MeV.

The evaluation of $\bar{E}_\beta$ presents certain problems. To calculate it, the shape of the β^--spectrum is needed, and this has been determined experimentally for a number of radioisotopes. Alternatively, it may be calculated from the theoretical shape of β-spectra, which in turn depends upon the maximum β-ray energy, the atomic number, and whether the transition is allowed or forbidden. Another approach is to measure it directly by calorimetric methods, and this method has been applied to a number of β-emitters in common use. For cases of allowed transitions, at low Z, $\bar{E}_\beta/E_{max}$ may be obtained analytically, and, for the range of β-particle energies encountered in radioactive decay, this quantity is found to lie in the range 0.4 ± 0.05. For forbidden transitions, and also for higher atomic numbers, the value may lie outside this range.

A few values for β-emitters with 100% of decays proceeding to 1 level (that is for radionuclides giving a single β-spectrum) are tabulated in Table 5.1.

Table 5.1

Mean β-particle energy, $\bar{E}_\beta$, for some β^--emitters emitting a single
β-spectrum (based on Spiers, 1968)

Isotope	Half-life	$E_\beta(\text{max})$ (MeV)	$\bar{E}_\beta$ (MeV)
^{3}H	12.3 y	0.018	0.006
^{14}C	5730 y	0.155	0.047
^{24}Na	15.0 h	1.39	0.55
^{32}P	14.3 d	1.71	0.694
^{35}S	87.4 d	0.167	0.049
^{45}Ca	164 d	0.254	0.076
^{82}Br	35.4 h	0.46	0.150
^{89}Sr	51 d	1.48	0.56
^{90}Sr	28 y	0.546	0.20
^{90}Y	64.2 h	2.28	0.93

If the activity in an organ is subject to exponential fall with time, due to decay or movement out of the compartment, the dose to a time T after administration may be obtained by integration

$$(D_\beta) = 5.92 \times 10^{-4} A_0 \bar{E}_\beta \int_0^T e^{-\lambda t}\, dt$$

$$= 5.92 \times 10^{-4} A_0 \bar{E}_\beta \frac{1}{\lambda}(1 - e^{-\lambda T}) \qquad (5.22)$$

where A_0 is the initial concentration of activity (in microcuries) and λ is the sum of the disintegration constant and the rate constant for loss from the compartment.

The dose to infinite time is often needed and is given by

$$(D_\beta)_\infty = 8.52 \times 10^{-4} A_0 \bar{E}_\beta T_{eff}, \qquad (5.23)$$

where T_{eff} is the effective half-life of the activity in the system (A_0 in μCi, $\bar{E}_\beta$ in MeV, T in seconds, $(D_\beta)_\infty$ in rads).

To take a simple example, we may evaluate the dose delivered by β-particles to the thyroid gland as a result of administration of a tracer dose of ^{131}I. Let the activity administered by 5 μCi. In patients with normal thyroid function, 25% of this is concentrated in the thyroid within a few hours of administration. Let the assumed mass of the gland be 20 g. The biological half-life for iodine in euthyroid subjects is about 70 days, and so (assuming a radioactive half-life of 8.05 days) the effective half-life may be calculated to be 7.2 days. Taking the mean β-ray energy of ^{131}I as 0.187 MeV, we may write

$$(D_\beta)_\infty(\text{rads}) = 8.52 \times 10^{-4} \times \frac{1.25}{20} \times 0.187 \times 7.2 \times 24 \times 3600$$

$$= \underline{6.20 \text{ rad}}$$

Although in the past such a dose has been regarded as acceptable in a diagnostic test, it is desirable to reduce it, and this may be done by using the 2.3 hr activity ^{132}I, with a mean β-ray energy of 0.49 MeV. D_∞ then becomes **215 mrad**. However, the time taken for ^{132}I to be concentrated is not short compared with the effective half-life (see Fig. 5.3) and the calculation must be refined, by integrating either analytically or graphically the curve for ^{132}I in that figure. An even smaller value for dose will be obtained. It is usual for the radiation dose using ^{132}I to be not more than about 1% of that which would result from the use of ^{131}I, for equal administered activities.

A further example may be drawn from pulmonary studies of the type described in section 5.8. The 'clearance' of oxygen–15 during breath-holding will be linear rather than exponential, but will be followed by an approximately exponential removal during subsequent washout. The clearance of a soluble gas such as CO_2 during breath-holding will however be exponential, and for purposes of calculating an absorbed radiation dose an exponential decline may be assumed. If we consider an inhaled activity of 1 mCi entering a lung of mass 1000 g, and an effective half-life τ seconds, we may write, taking $\bar{E}_\beta = 0.72$ MeV,

$$D_\beta(\text{in rads}) = 8.52 \times 10^{-4} \times \frac{10^3}{1000} \times 0.72 \times \tau \,(\text{seconds}).$$

For examples for an effective half-life in the lung, of 30 seconds, we get $D_\beta = 18.4$ **mrad**.

Retention times may be longer if washout is prolonged, but the effective half-life can of course never exceed the radioactive half-life of 130 s. Such radiation doses are normally acceptable in diagnostic tests, and a series of 4 or 5 measurements, each involving inspiration of 1 mCi of ^{15}O-labelled oxygen or carbon dioxide, imparts a radiation dose no higher than that which is associated with many diagnostic x-ray radiographic examinations.

If charged-particle equilibrium does not apply, more explicit expressions for the dose (or dose-rate) as function of distance from a source have to be obtained. For β-radiation, the 'point-source' distribution function may be used. This may be expressed as

$$D_\beta = \frac{K e^{-vx}}{(vx)^2} \tag{5.24}$$

where x is the distance from the source, and K is a constant depending upon the medium, the β-ray energy and the source activity. v is an 'effective' absorption coefficient of the medium for the radiation, and is an empirical quantity based on the observation that the loss of β-particles from a beam varies approximately exponentially with thickness, if the β-spectrum is continuous and is of the form usually observed in β-decay.

To obtain consistency with experimental measurements, Loevinger proposed a 'two-part' function

$$\left.\begin{aligned} D_1 &= \frac{K}{(vx)^2} & vx \leqslant 1 \\[2mm] D_2 &= \frac{K}{(vx)} e^{-(vx-1)} & vx > 1 \end{aligned}\right\} \tag{5.25}$$

which falls less rapidly than (5.24), particularly at higher values of (vx).

In order to apply these methods to obtain, for example, the dose rate near the surface of the organ containing the radioactivity, where charged-particle equilibrium would not be expected to exist, detailed calculations are needed, based on integration of the point-source function (5.24), the two-part function (5.25) or other more elaborate functions of the type described by Loevinger (1956), and discussed by, for example, Spiers (1968). As an example, consider the β-radiation dose within, but near the surface of, a sphere containing a uniform distribution of radioactivity. For a large sphere the dose rate will be uniform throughout most of its volume. At points within a distance of order $1/v$ from the surface, charged particle equilibrium will no longer obtain, and the dose (or dose rate) will become progressively less than the dose at the centre, falling to a value of approximately 50% at the surface. If the radius of the sphere is not large in comparison with $1/v$, charged particle equilibrium will not be achieved anywhere within the sphere, and the dose at the centre will itself be less than the equilibrium value.

When considering doses from internal β-emitters, a major difficulty arises because of non-uniform take-up of the labelled substances. Pursuing the example of iodine uptake in the thyroid, this has been shown by autoradiography of excised samples to be extremely non-uniform, and the maximum doses associated with 'hot-spots' have been shown to be as much as 80 times the mean value. Theoretical work has been carried out on the dose distributions to be expected from small spherical volumes distributed on a regular lattice, which supports the view that large variations of dose within the gland are to be expected. This had led to the realisation that β-particles of higher energy, or x-rays from isotopes decaying by electron capture, might lead to improvements brought about by a more uniform dose distribution, and in this connection the use of the positron emitting isotope ^{124}I ($E_{max} = 2.15$ MeV) has been reported by Phillips (1957), and its dosimetric aspects discussed by Matthews and Fowler (1960).

An important dosimetric problem is the calculation of the dose to the bone marrow resulting from β-emitters trapped in mineral bone. The fission product ^{90}Sr remains in bone for very long periods, and the range of the β-particles from the radioactive daughter ^{90}Y is sufficient to enter the erythropoietic tissue in the marrow, where it represents a radiological hazard. One method of approaching this problem is to use the point dose functions (5.24, 5.25) to obtain estimates of the dose from β-emitters of different geometrical forms (for example distributed along surfaces). A further use of point dose functions is in connection with calculation of the radiation dose from insoluble radioactive particles which may be inhaled and become lodged essentially permanently in the lung. The point dose function affords a method of calculating the β-radiation dose rate at the surface of particles of different radii, and can be used to assess the radiological hazards of radioactive dust and other air-borne particles.

Dosimetry associated with γ-radiation from internal radioisotopes is made difficult by the fact that the mean free path is normally several centimetres, which implies that a simple approach based on equilibrium concepts cannot be adopted. If however, the activity is concentrated in a relatively small region, and the dose to other parts of the body requires to be calculated, the expression

$$D_\gamma = \frac{A\Gamma}{x^2} e^{-\mu x} \tag{5.26}$$

may be used. Γ is the specific gamma emission discussed in section 4.8, and A the activity. The quantity μ in this expression is normally not known precisely – the total attenuation coefficient is not an appropriate value to use, because the scattered radiation produced by the Compton effect remains in the system. A value for μ equal to the attenuation coefficient minus the Compton scattering coefficient may be used, or alternatively a 'build-up factor', increasing with distance from the source, as used in calculations of radiation shielding in 'broad-beam' conditions, may be practicable.

The effect of γ-ray dose within an organ is usually small compared with that associated with β-radiation, because much of the γ-radiation will escape; but this will not always be so, for example, in the case of ^{99m}Tc (when the β-radiation is only that associated with internal conversion) or electron capture isotopes (where the x-rays will have a mean free path intermediate between β-radiation and γ-particles). The γ-ray dose within a uniformly activated sphere may be calculated analytically, if self-absorption is neglected in the sense that the dose rate at a distance x is taken as $D_\gamma = \Gamma/x^2$, without an exponential term. For a concentration C of activity, the dose at the centre of a sphere of radius R may be calculated by integration to be (referring to Fig. 5.17)

$$D_\gamma = 4\pi\Gamma CR \tag{5.27}$$

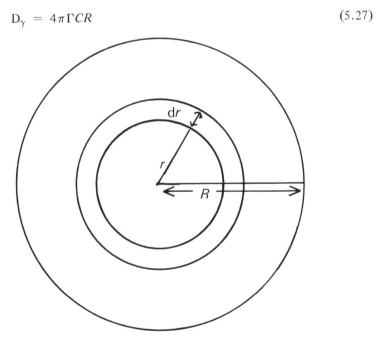

Fig. 5.17   Illustrating calculation of dose at the centre of a sphere of uniform activity

At a distance r from the centre, and writing $r/R = a$, the dose may be shown to be

$$D_\gamma = 4\pi\Gamma CR \left(\frac{1}{2} + \frac{1-a^2}{4a} \ln \frac{1+a}{|1-a|} \right) \tag{5.28}$$

inside and outside the sphere.

At the surface of the sphere the dose is one-half of the dose at the centre. It has also been shown (Mayneord, 1950) that the mean dose throughout the whole sphere is three-quarters of the dose at the centre. This result enables the average dose throughout an organ containing uniform activity to be estimated.

Although the contribution from γ-radiation to the radiation dose in an organ containing radioactivity may be small compared with that due to the β-radiation, the whole body dose from γ-radiation may nevertheless require estimation. Furthermore, in the case of ^{24}Na, which becomes distributed throughout the body in the extracellular fluid, the γ-radiation is responsible for 80% of the total absorbed dose, and so requires to be calculated in tracer studies involving this radioisotope.

The dosimetry of internally absorbed γ-emitters may be developed in a formal manner by the use of the Reciprocal Dose Theorem, which states that the dose delivered to a point from a uniform volume distribution of activity is equal to the average absorbed dose delivered to that volume by the same amount of activity concentrated at that point. This may be established by writing, for the dose delivered to a point from an amount of activity A distributed uniformly throughout a volume V, and referring to Fig. 5.18,

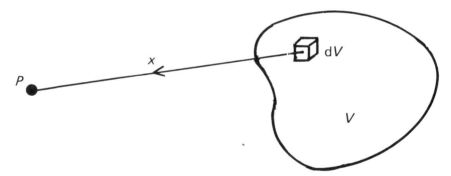

Fig. 5.18 Illustrating the Reciprocal Dose Theorem

$$D_\gamma = \int_v \frac{\Gamma}{x^2} \frac{A}{V} e^{-\mu x} \, dv \qquad (5.29)$$

If we now concentrate the activity A at point P, it may be seen that the integral dose (that is total energy deposited in the volume V) is given by

$$I_\gamma = A \int_v \frac{\Gamma}{x^2} e^{-\mu x} \, dv \qquad (5.30)$$

and the average dose is equal to this quantity divided by V, which is the same as (5.29).

Corollaries of this theorem (using the form given by Wagner, 1968) state that (a) 2 sources containing the same total activity deliver to each other the same **average** absorbed dose irrespective of size, shape, or distance.
(b) Two sources with the same **concentration** of activity deliver to each other the same integral absorbed dose irrespective of size, shape, and distance.

The theorem is thus able to facilitate calculations of the effect of a distributed source of activity on neighbouring organs, and particularly the mutal effects of two distributed sources.

The internal dosimetry of α-radiation has been left until last because, in a sense, it is simpler than the internal dosimetry of β- and γ-radiation. α-particles are of such short range that the mean dose to even a small organism, or small region of tissue, can be derived simply by evaluating the emitted energy (that is, number of alpha particles $\times$ particle energy), and dividing by the mass. In the case of irradiation in a very restricted region (that is, a region which is small compared even with the range of α-particles), the Bethe–Bloch formula can be used to obtain the energy loss per unit thickness traversed, which can be related to macroscopic dose if the mass thickness of the material (for example cell preparation) is known. It will be appreciated however, that the macroscopic dose does not convey much about the energy deposition on a cellular scale, which will normally be the important feature of the absorption of energy from internal α-emitters. The propotion of energy deposited by δ-rays for example may be required to be known, and this may be obtained from calculations based on the Bethe–Bloch expression. The deposition of energy in soft tissue from α-particles originating in bone is a dosimetric problem which may be approached using the Bethe–Bloch expression, and is a problem of practical importance in connection with the long-term effects of α-emitters ingested and deposited in the skeleton, giving rise to α-irradiation of the marrow. The dosimetry of α-emitting radioactive dust particles may be approached in a similar manner.

FURTHER READING

Atkins, G. L. (1969) *Multicompartment models in biological systems* Methuen
Belcher, E. H. and Vetter, H. (Eds.) (1971) *Radioisotopes in Medical Diagnosis* Butterworth
Spiers, F. W. (1968) *Radioisotopes in the Human Body* Academic Press
Wagner, H. N. (Ed.) (1968) *Principles of Nuclear Medicine* Saunders

REFERENCES

Anger, H. O (1964) *J. Nucl. Med.*, **5**, 515
Bigler, R. E., Laughlin, J. S., Davies, R. Jr. and Evans, J. C. (1976) *Radiation Res.*, **67**, 266

Burch, P. R. J. (1962) in *Whole Body Counting,* IAEA Vienna, 425

Clarke, J. C. and Buckingham, P. D. (1975) *Short-lived radioactive gases for clinical use* Butterworths

Dollery, C. T., Dyson, N. A. and Sinclair, J. D. (1960) *Journ. App. Physiol.,* **15**, 411

Dolphin, G. W. and Eve, I. S. (1963) *Phys. Med. Biol.,* **8**, 193

Dyson, N. A., Hugh-Jones, P., Newbery, G. R., Sinclair, J. D. and West, J. B. (1960) *Brit. Med. Journ.,* **1**, 231

Dyson, N. A. (1960) *Phys. Med. Biol.,* **4**, 376

Edelman, I. S. and Liebman, J. (1959) *Amer. J. Med.,* **27**, 256

Jones, T., Clark, J. C., Hughes, J. M. and Rosenzweig, D. Y. (1970) *J. Nucl. Med.,* **11**, 118

Leach, M. O., Bell, C. M. J., Thomas, B. J., Dabek, J. T., James, H. M., Chettle, D. R. and Fremlin, J. H. (1978) *Phys. Med. Biol.,* **23**, 282

Loevinger, R., Japha, E. M. and Brownell, G. L. (1956) in *Radiation Dosimetry* (Eds. Hine, G. J. and Brownell, G. L., Chapter 16) Academic Press

Mallard, J. R. (1971) see Belcher, E. H. and Vetter, H. (Eds.) in Further Reading, above

Matthews, C. M. E. (1964) *Brit. J. Radiol.* **37**, 531

Matthews, C. M. E (1971) see Belcher, E. H. and Vetter, H. (Eds.) in Further Reading, above

Matthews, C. M. E. and Fowler, J. F. (1960) *Nature,* **186**, 983

Mayneord, W. V. (1950) *Brit. J. Radiol.* (suppl. No. 2)

Phillips, A. F. (1957) *Brit. J. Radiol.,* **30**, 247

Silver, S. (1962) *Radioactive isotopes in medicine and biology* Kimpton

Sweet, W. H., Mealey, J. Jr., Brownell, G. L. and Aronow, S. (1959) in *Medical Radioisotope Scanning* IAEA Vienna

Trott, N. G. (1971) see Belcher, E. H. and Vetter, H. (Eds.) in Further Reading, above

West, J. B. (1963) *Brit. Med. Bull.,* **19**, 53

Yano, Y., McRae, J., and Anger, H. O. (1970) *J. Nucl. Med.,* **11**, 674

CHAPTER 6

Neutrons in biology and clinical medicine

6.1 INTERACTIONS WITH MATTER

In Chapter 1 we discussed the interactions between charged particles and matter, and saw that these depend primarily on the Coulomb forces between the incident particles and the electrons and nuclei in the material undergoing bombardment. When considering the interactions between neutrons and matter, we note immediately that the uncharged nature of the neutron means that Coulomb forces are absent; in its most elementary form, interaction with matter depends upon the 'hard sphere' property of a neutron, that is, upon the repulsive force exerted between nucleons in a close encounter. These 'billiard-ball type' collisions are an important interaction mechanism and take place essentially with atomic nuclei rather than with orbital electrons. Also of importance is the attractive force between nucleons, which ensures a finite probability that a neutron will be captured, especially when the neutron energy is low. This capture results in the release of binding energy in the form of γ-radiation. Such radiative capture processes have already been referred to in Chapter 2.

Although the collision processes referred to above are analogous to classical collisions between hard spheres, they are modified by the wave nature of the neutron, so that diffraction effects can appear, modifying for example the angular distribution of emitted particles of scattered neutrons. This becomes important at energies above a few MeV, but the classical collision processes nevertheless help to establish an initial understanding of neutron interactions.

6.1.1 Elastic scattering

At energies where the 'hard sphere' approach may be used, the behaviour of the neutron and the struck nucleus is determined by the conservation laws. If we consider the case of a 'head-on' collision (Fig. 6.1) we may write

$$m_1 v_1 = m_2 v_2 + m_1 v_1'$$

and $$m_1 v_1^2 = m_2 v_2^2 + m_1 v_1'^2$$

from conservation of momentum and energy respectively.

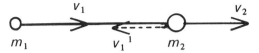

Fig. 6.1 Collision at zero impact parameter between neutron and nucleus

Hence we may establish that

$$E' = E \left(\frac{A-1}{A+1}\right)^2 \tag{6.1}$$

Where E and E' are respectively the neutron energies before and after the collision, and A the mass number of the struck nucleus. For heavy nuclei, the neutron energy is changed little, whereas for a hydrogen nucleus the whole of the energy is transferred, and the neutron comes to rest.

For collisions which are not head-on, the energy change is less, and it can be shown that, if an average over all impact parameters is taken, the mean neutron energy after the collision is midway between the incident energy and that given by (6.1)

$$\bar{E}' = \frac{E+E'}{2} = E.\frac{A^2+1}{(A+1)^2} \tag{6.2}$$

Energy is thus transferred to the medium, and the nuclei which are set in motion will lose their energy by the processes described in sections 1.1–1.6. This is the essential feature of energy absorption from a neutron beam, because the struck atoms invariably lose some orbital electrons thereby becoming ionized, if the neutron energy exceeds the binding energy of the outer electrons.

The slowing down, or 'moderation', of neutrons by elastic collisions is an essential feature of the 'thermal' nuclear reactor, in which the fission process can occur with adequately high cross-section only if the neutrons already released in fission have been slowed down sufficiently to achieve thermal equilibrium with their surroundings. Such thermal neutrons have an energy distribution given by the relation

$$N(E) = \text{const.} \frac{E}{(kT)^2} e^{-E/kT} \tag{6.3}$$

The neutron spectrum is now dependent on the temperature of the medium. Elastic collisions will impart insufficient energy to ionize the atoms. No further deposition of energy within the medium can occur, and the neutron may survive many further collisions before capture. Typical times are $10\,\mu s$ for the slowing down of a 10 MeV neutron to thermal energies, and a further $100\,\mu s$ before capture takes place in a hydrogenous medium. If the latter consists of deuterium, the diffusion time after thermalisation may be much longer, because of the very low capture cross-section of deuterium for slow neutrons.

6.1.2 Neutron capture

When capture occurs, an energy equal to the binding energy per nucleon (Fig. 2.1) becomes available, normally as γ-radiation. The spectrum of γ-radiation depends on the structure of the product nucleus; normally there will be several lines in the spectrum, except in the case of certain light elements in which the levels are widely spaced, giving rise to only one photon energy. Examples of this are $^{14}N(n,\gamma)^{15}N$, which is accompanied by a single line of 10.8 MeV energy, and $H(n,\gamma)^2D$, in which the emitted γ-ray has an energy of 2.3 MeV, which is anomalously low because of the loosely-bound nature of the deuteron.

Radiative capture is the usual fate of a neutron, and the γ-radiation thus produced will contribute to the radiation dose absorbed by the medium from the beam. In one or two instances, neutron capture is followed by particle emission, for example in the $^{10}B(n,\alpha)^7Li$ reaction, where the compound nucleus ^{11}B is unstable against particle emission, and disintegrates into an α-particle and a ^7Li nucleus.

Radiative capture cross-sections for thermal neutrons vary widely, from less than a millibarn for capture in deuterium to 10^3–10^4 barn for capture in cadmium (2550 barn for the natural mixture of isotopes) or gadolinium (46000 barn). Capture cross-sections for thermal neutrons lie typically in the range 1–10 barns; they may vary in a simple manner that is according to the $1/v$ law, or may have resonances of the Breit–Wigner type superimposed.

6.1.3 Inelastic scattering

When a fast neutron is scattered, it may leave the scattering nucleus in an excited state. The neutron then travels with reduced energy, and the nucleus subsequently deexcites with the emission of γ-radiation. Cross-sections for this process tend to be small, but may nevertheless be significant. For example, when shielding materials are being used in mixed neutron and γ-radiation fields, the occurrence of inelastic neutron scattering in the γ-ray shielding materials can contribute to the γ-radiation already present in the system.

6.1.4 Fission, Spallation and other nuclear processes

Many heavy nuclei are, in principle, unstable against fission, and we have already illustrated (Fig. 2.11) the spontaneous fission probability as a function of the parameter Z^2/A. Nuclei for which the probability of spontaneous fission is low or zero can nevertheless have fission induced in them by charged particles, or by fast neutron bombardment, when the energy introduced may be sufficient to overcome the 'fission barrier'. The existence of this barrier may be understood when it is realised that, in order to initiate the fission process, a nucleus must be deformed into an ellipsoidal form, against the attractive force between nucleons. This process will normally require an input of energy. At a later stage in the fission process the two fragments will become separated and will fly apart by Coulomb repulsion, the energy for this process being made available by the stronger binding of the nucleons in the fragments (see Fig. 2.1). Fast neutrons can therefore be absorbed by certain heavy elements, and energy is therefore released by the fission process, the amount being usually of the order of 200 MeV. The fission fragments are highly ionized, and produce dense ionization tracks in the medium. They are also radioactive, because of the high neutron-to-proton ratio, and deposit further amounts of energy by the normal processes of nuclear decay.

In addition to the fission fragments, two or three neutrons are also released in the fission process. The energy of these is of the order of 1 MeV each, and is distributed according to the spectrum illustrated in Fig. 6.2.

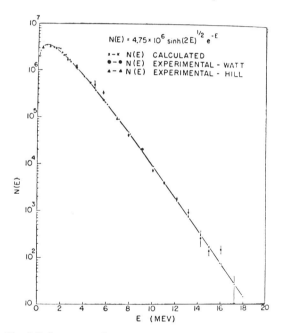

Fig. 6.2 Spectrum of neutrons released in fission (Watt, 1952)

To achieve fission, energy sufficient to overcome the fission barrier has to be introduced. Many heavy elements are fissionable by fast neutrons. For example, the thresholds for fission in ^{238}U and ^{209}Bi are 1.5 MeV and ~50 MeV respectively. However, in a few cases, fission can be induced by thermal neutrons, that is, the binding energy alone of the incoming neutron is sufficient. The nuclei in which this can occur are ^{233}U, ^{235}U and ^{239}Pu. The neutrons released in fission will then have sufficient energy to cause further fissions, and a nuclear chain reaction can be achieved, if the system is greater than a certain critical size.

To control the reaction, neutron absorbers have to be introduced into the system, and a steady state then becomes possible. This is the principle on which the nuclear reactor is based. The isotopes listed above are rather specialised – the ^{235}U occurs in natural uranium only to the extent of 1 part in 140, and the others do not occur in nature, although can be made artificially. It is practicable, however, to make a reactor using natural uranium, providing that a moderator is incorporated which ensures that the neutrons produced in fission are slowed down to the point at which the absorption of neutrons by non-fissioning processes (for example absorption in ^{238}U) is not sufficiently serious to prevent the maintenance of a chain reaction by means of fission in the ^{235}U isotope. The moderator has to reduce the neutron energy by a sizeable fraction at each elastic collision, and must have a very small capture cross-section. Suitable materials, for use with natural uranium, are graphite or heavy water. If the uranium is enriched in ^{235}U, the conditions regarding the moderator are relaxed, and ordinary water may be used. These systems form the basis of nuclear power programmes currently under development in many countries.

Fast neutrons can also cause fragmentation of nuclei (including the detachment of several neutrons) if the energy is sufficiently high, that is 50 MeV or more. This process is called **spallation**, and is becoming increasingly interesting in view of the drive towards higher energy neutrons for radiotherapy and because of the possibility of extending the range of radioisotopes produced by nuclear reactions.

Finally, it should be mentioned that other types of nuclear reaction can also take place when beams of neutrons interact with matter. This aspect has been referred to briefly in section 2.2, in connection with the production of isotopes using reactions induced by either fast or slow neutrons. So far as biological and medical aspects of neutron physics are concerned, two examples may be mentioned here. First, the ^{10}B(n,α)^{7}Li reaction is important because it is the basis of several types of slow neutron detector. The reaction follows a $1/v$ law, and the cross-section has a value of 3820 barn for thermal neutrons at room temperature, or 755 barn for the naturally-occurring mixture of isotopes. If the boron is used as a gaseous compound such as boron trifluoride, it may be used in an ionization chamber or proportional counter, in which case a signal is produced by the α-particle and the recoiling ^{7}Li nucleus. ^{10}B is present in natural boron to the extent of 18.5%, and so is an abundant isotope, readily available either as natural boron or as a separated isotope (see section 6.4.2).

The second example is the ^{14}N(n,p)^{14}C reaction. This occurs as a result of continuous production in the upper atmosphere, as a consequence of the presence of neutrons produced by the cosmic radiation, and is responsible for the presence in living matter of small but measurable amounts of this radioisotope. Its continued presence in dead biological material (for example wood), decaying with its half-life of 5,700 years, has enabled a method of archaeological dating to be developed. The same reaction is also used in the nuclear reactor for the preparation of ^{14}C in concentrated form for incorporation in a wide variety of organic compounds for use in research.

Both these examples are reactions caused by slow neutrons.

6.1.5 Energy-loss and linear energy transfer

The treatment of the rate of energy loss of charged particles in Chapter 1 enables us to obtain values for the quantity $dE/d(\rho x)$, either by calculation from the Bethe–Bloch expression, or from the extensive tabulations which now exist. The energy loss dE/dx, expressed in units of energy per unit length, is readily obtained from this, and is of great importance when the manner of transference of energy to matter is under consideration. In the context of this book, the concept of radiation dose may be readily understood in macroscopic terms as being the energy deposited per unit mass, in water, biological tissue, or some other medium. On considering the mechanisms underlying the response of biological material to radiation, however it soon becomes apparent that a more detailed examination of the physical processes is required, before the biological processes can be considered.

The energy loss per unit path length is known as the linear energy transfer, or LET. For an electron set in motion by the absorption of a γ-ray photon this is typically in the region of 0.2–0.5 keV $(\mu m)^{-1}$, and in a practical situation the electrons so released will extend over a continuous range of energies, as will readily be understood from an examination of the several interactions which may take place between γ-rays and matter. Low energy electrons set in motion by, for example, 100 kVp x-rays will have a somewhat higher LET than those released by the absorption of γ-rays from ^{60}Co or radium.

The mechanisms for neutron absorption will normally set heavy particles (for example protons or atomic nuclei) in motion, and it will be clear that the LET for these particles is of a much higher order of magnitude than for electrons. For a 1 MeV proton, dE/dx in biological tissue is approximately 20 keV $(\mu m)^{-1}$, and for α-particles and other light nuclei the LET is even greater. The differences in the biological effects of different radiations, for a given absorbed dose, are attributable in principle to the very substantial differences in the mechanisms, at the microscopic level, of energy deposition. In particular, the energy deposited in an individual biological cell will depend strongly on the LET of the radiation and the structure of the track of ionization left by the moving charge. This last point may now be examined in more detail.

Ionization takes place mainly by the transfer of small amounts of energy in the course of the slowing down process. Occasionally, however, an atomic electron will be ejected with substantial energy sufficient to produce its own track. This is the so-called δ-ray. Such tracks may be seen by cloud chamber techniques or by photographic emulsions. The important point is that the energy used in the production of a δ-ray is not deposited at the point of production, but is distributed along the path of the δ-ray. It does not therefore contribute to the local deposition of energy, although it makes its contribution to the total energy loss of the moving charged particles. The 'local' LET is therefore **less** than the total LET, by an amount depending on the fraction of energy converted to δ-rays. These δ-rays must therefore be regarded as separate tracks for purposes of calculating the local LET, and it is conventional to treat all δ-rays of 100 eV or more as being separate tracks, and to designate the local LET as LET_{100}.

The fraction of energy converted into δ-rays may be considerable. This is illustrated by some calculations of Burch (1957a) who evaluated the ratio of LET_{100} to LET_{total} for electrons of various kinetic energies. Representative values from his table are given in Table 6.1. The ratio is substantially less than 1 throughout most of the table.

Table 6.1

Fraction of energy deposited locally by electrons, as a function of electron kinetic energy† (after Burch, 1957a)

Electron kinetic energy	$\dfrac{LET_{100}}{LET_{total}}$
keV	
0.05	1.00
0.175	1.00
0.35	0.933
1.4	0.752
5.6	0.675
22.4	0.631
89.6	0.602
358.4	0.578
MeV	
1.434	0.551
5.735	0.505
22.94	0.419

† Burch groups the electrons into a number of ranges of kinetic energy. Only the median values of his energy ranges are given here.

A further consequence of δ-ray production is that much of the energy deposited in a medium is deposited by electrons of relatively low energy, for which the LET is in fact *higher* than both the mean and the local values along the main track. In order fully to express this, it is necessary to determine, either experimentally or by calculation, the spectrum of charged particles set in motion by a given incident radiation spectrum (of photons, electrons, or heavy particles), and then to calculate the fraction of energy deposited in the medium per unit interval of LET throughout the whole relevant range of LET_{100} values. Burch (1957b) has presented data from which the LET spectrum for various sources of radiation may be calculated. The LET spectrum associated with an incident beam of ^{60}Co γ-rays is seen (Fig. 6.3) to extend over a wide range of values.

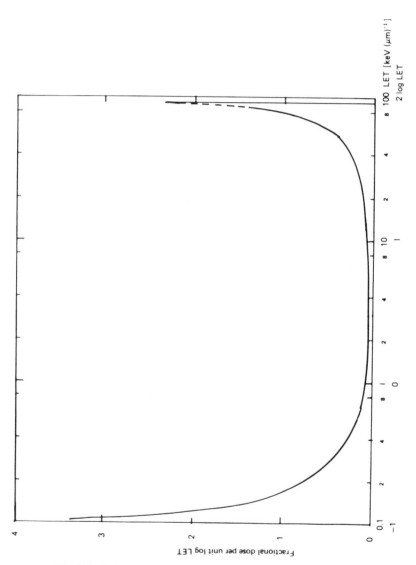

Fig. 6.3 LET spectrum for the electrons released in water by ^{60}Co γ-rays (calculated from the data of Burch, 1957b)

It has peaks in two widely-separated regions of the spectrum, one corresponding to the local LET along the main tracks, and the other corresponding mainly to the ends of the subsidiary tracks of the δ-rays. It is clear that only when an LET spectrum has been obtained is one in a position to analyse the nature and extent of radiobiological damage at the cellular level.

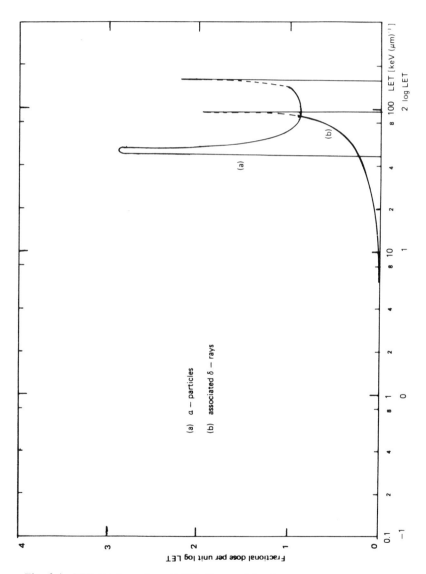

Fig. 6.4   LET spectrum from 5.3 MeV α-particles (calculated from the data of Burch, 1957b)

Turning to the LET spectrum from neutrons, it will be appreciated that much (though not all) of the energy is deposited by densely ionizing particles. In biological tissue, about 85% of the energy is transferred by recoil protons, and an LET_{100} can be calculated for this as a function of proton energy. If the incident neutron spectrum is known, the proton spectrum can be derived, and the LET_{100} spectrum obtained from this. An example of an LET spectrum from α-particles and associated δ-rays is illustrated in Fig. 6.4.

The differences between γ-radiation and neutrons are further intensified by presence of even more densely ionizing tracks from nuclear recoils. Nuclear reactions involving break-up of the ^{12}C nucleus make only a small contribution in the case of the neutron beams which have hitherto been available for radio-biological and radiotherapeutic work (section 6.3), but if neutrons of higher energy are used, nuclear reactions, including spallation, become more significant, thereby enhancing the high LET regions of the LET spectrum. We shall see in section 6.3 that there is reason to believe that this would be an advantage in these fields.

6.2 PRODUCTION OF NEUTRONS

6.2.1 Laboratory neutron sources

Laboratory sources of neutrons have been available for many years and are usually based upon the combination of an α-emitter and a light element, in intimate mixture within a single capsule. Historically, radium in equilibrium with its daughter products has been used, because its α-spectrum (extending up to 4.8 MeV) is suitable for the bombardment of beryllium in order to produce fast neutrons by the (α, n) reaction, which in beryllium (100% ^9Be) has a Q value of $+5.7$ MeV. Neutrons with energies up to about 10 MeV are therefore released. Early difficulties in ensuring reproducible neutron output were approached first by combining radium and beryllium in the same crystal lattice, and subsequently by very careful mixing of radium with finely-divided beryllium powder. The mixture is doubly encapsulated in a stainless steel cylinder. The yield of neutrons from such a source is included in Table 6.2.

Radium (with its decay products) has a high output of γ-radiation which may be a disadvantage in some applications. It has long been superseded by polonium–210 and, more recently, americum–241; the long half-life of the latter enables essentially permanent sources to be manufactured.

Other α-emitter/target combinations in current use as laboratory neutron sources are listed in Table 6.2.

An example of a fast neutron spectrum from an (α, n) laboratory source is illustrated in Fig. 6.5.

It is usually necessary to reduce the amount of background γ-radiation to a minimum, and in this respect the choice of light element is as important as the choice of the primary α-emitter. For example, boron rather than beryllium has sometimes been preferred on account of the lower level of γ-radiation produced by the (α, n) reaction on boron.

Table 6.2
Yields of neutron sources

		Half-life	n s^{-1} Ci^{-1}	γ-emission mR h^{-1} at 1 metre from a source of 10^6 n s^{-1}	Neutron energy (MeV)	
					Mean	Maximum
(α,n) sources with Beryllium target	Americium–241	458 y	2.7×10^6	<0.1	~ 6	11
	Polonium–210	138.4 d	2.5×10^6	0.04	4.3	10.8
	Radium–226 (+ daughters)	1620 y	1.3×10^7	60		
(α,n) source with Boron target	Polonium–210	138.4 d	0.2×10^6			5.0
(γ,n) sources with Beryllium target	Radium–226 (+ daughters)	1620 y	1.3×10^6			0.7
	Antimony–124	60 d	1.6×10^6			0.0248
Spontaneous fission source	Californium–252	2.65 y	2.3×10^{12} (neutrons per gram per second)		Fission spectrum;	

Data reproduced mainly from *The Radiochemical Manual*, (1966)

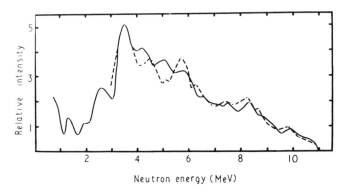

Fig. 6.5 Neutron spectrum from an americium–beryllium (α,n) laboratory source. (Hannan *et al.*,1973. The dashed curve was measured at the Radiochemical Centre, Amersham)

Neutron sources based on (γ,n) reactions are occasionally used. A Ra–Be (γ,n) source can be prepared by surrounding a radium tube (for example 4–5 mm in diameter $\times$ 5 cm in length) with a cylinder of beryllium metal. Although the background of γ-radiation is necessarily high, the system has the advantage that the neutrons can be 'switched off' by removing the beryllium, so that the response to γ-radiation of the physical or chemical system under study, can be measured separately, and corrected for. A neutron source for specialised application is the (γ,n) source using ^{124}Sb as the γ-ray emitter and beryllium as the target material. This has been used in nuclear reactors in circumstances where a permanent neutron source for start-up procedures is required. The neutrons produced have an intermediate energy of about 30 keV (^{124}Sb $\gamma = 1.71$ MeV; photoneutron threshold of Be $= 1.68$ MeV) and the source, which is prepared by the (n,γ) reaction on antimony metal, is continuously reactivated during reactor operation.

The remaining type of laboratory neutron source is that based on spontaneous fission. We have seen how certain heavy isotopes undergo fission spontaneously, and that the disintegration constant for this process rises with increase of the parameter Z^2/A. For elements of $Z \gtrsim 96$ the process contributes significantly to the radioactive decay of the nuclide, (which is usually predominately by α-emission) and in the case of ^{252}Cf the process is sufficiently probable ($\approx 3\%$ of disintegrations) to create a high yield of neutrons, the half-life being long enough (2.6 y) to facilitate the preparation of semi-permanent sources using this material. The spectrum is of lower energy than the (α,n) sources described earlier.

6.2.2 Nuclear reactors

The process of nuclear fission has been described elsewhere in this book (sections 2.5, 6.1.4) and we have seen how the neutrons released in fission may be used to maintain a controlled chain reaction in an assembly consisting of fissile material, moderator, coolant, and control rods. A reactor therefore constitutes an abundant supply of slow and fast neutrons. These neutrons are available within the core of the reactor and may be used to activate small samples placed there. Fluxes of thermal neutrons up to 10^{15} $(cm)^{-2} s^{-1}$ may be obtained near the centre of a high flux reactor, although the flux falls off near the periphery, and values two or three orders-of-magnitude lower are more usual in neutron activation procedures.

In radiobiological work we are concerned mainly with the fluxes and beams available externally. Fig. 6.6 illustrates an arrangement by which several beams may be made available. A beam line 'looking' at the core will allow a fission spectrum of neutrons to escape, and a flux of the order of 10^{10} $(cm)^{-2} s^{-1}$ is available.

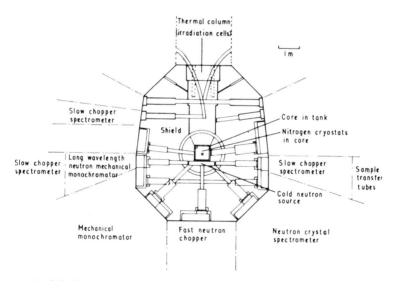

Fig. 6.6 Illustrating the beams available from the HERALD research reactor
(Walker 1967)

If a graphite column passes through the biological shield surrounding the reactor core, thermal neutrons will diffuse outwards, and fluxes of order of $10^{6} (cm)^{-2} s^{-1}$ are by this means made available in an experimental area adjacent to the reactor. Such 'thermal columns' are widely used for experimental work.

6.2.3 Accelerator sources of neutrons

The nuclear reactions discussed in Chapter 2 provide the principal methods of producing beams of fast neutrons for experimental research and for clinical use in neutron therapy and *in vivo* activation analysis. The (d,n) reaction is the most frequently used, with a light element as target. Neutrons are produced either by direct interaction, or by 'stripping' and the yield is high enough to make this reaction attractive. The Q value of the ^{9}Be (d,n) reaction is 4 MeV, hence if 15 MeV deuterons are used or a thick target, a continuous spectrum of fast neutrons is generated up to a high energy limit of 19 MeV, down to an energy determined essentially by the coulomb barrier between projectile and target nucleus. The low energy limit will be in the region of 6 MeV. The Lithium (p,n) reaction may also be used. The main problems in producing fast neutron beams by this method are concerned with obtaining adequate dissipation of power at the target. Oil cooling or water cooling are normally used to facilitate this, and a rotating target may be used to reduce the maximum surface temperature to which the target is subjected. For much radiobiological work neutrons produced by these reactions are to be preferred to unmoderated fission neutrons because of their higher energy and penetration.

Other reactions used for neutron production consist of the fusion reactions

$$D + D \rightarrow {}^3He + n + 3.5 \, MeV$$

and $$D + T \rightarrow {}^4He + n + 17.6 \, MeV$$

These exothermic reactions will proceed readily with quite low beam energies, and deuterons of a few hundred keV will produce a good yield of neutrons. In the case of the DT reactions the tritium is absorbed on to a metal foil, and the reaction produces neutrons of about 14 MeV, which are widely used in applied radiation work. Sealed-off tubes are available in which deuterium or a mixture of deuterium and tritium is ionized and accelerated. A yield of 10^{12} neutrons per second is quoted by one manufacturer, for an electrical rating of 250 kV and 30 mA. Such tubes are currently undergoing evaluation for use in neutron therapy.

6.3 NEUTRONS IN RADIOBIOLOGY AND RADIOTHERAPY

In order to appreciate the special role which neutrons play in radiobiological and radiotherapeutic research, we must first consider the nature of the response of biological material to ionizing radiation.

The results of irradiation are most simply understood if we consider a very simple biological system, such as a virus preparation. These can be subjected to doses of x-radiation at various levels, and the fraction of viruses surviving irradiation at a particular dose can be plotted against that dose. An example of the results of such an experiment is illustrated in Fig. 6.7. The graph is exponential in form. This suggests a simple model for radiation action, as follows: If a virus is inactivated by a single interaction with the incident radiation, we can write, for the number dN of viruses inactivated by a dose increment dD,

$$dN = -Nk\,dD$$

When integrated this leads directly to the equation

$$N = N_0 e^{-kD} \tag{6.1}$$

for the survival following a dose D. This is observed in practice which suggests the validity of a 'single-hit' or 'target' theory of virus inactivation. By considering the number of ion-pairs formed by a dose of radiation, and making certain assumptions about the number of pairs in each 'cluster' of ion-pairs, it is possible to elaborate the theory to a point at which an effective target volume for inactivation can be derived, and it appears that one such interaction, anywhere within the virus, is sufficient to cause inactivation. The dose leading to 37% survival is known as the inactivation dose or 'mean lethal dose', and is obtained by setting D equal to $1/k$.

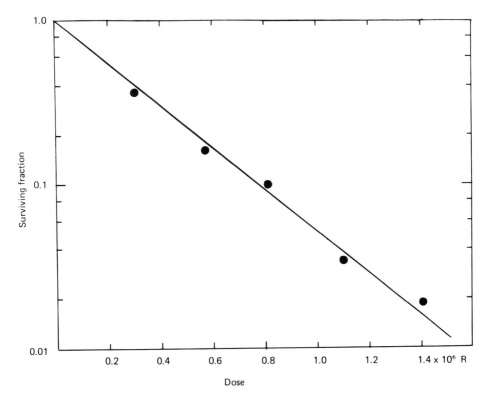

Fig. 6.7 Survival curve for irradiated plant virus (γ-rays on potato virus X, Lea, 1955)

For mammalian cells the situation is not quite so straight-forward. The survival curve takes the form illustrated in Fig. 6.8. Let us set up a more general theory, using as a basis the hypothesis that n independent interactions are necessary to cause inactivation of a cell.

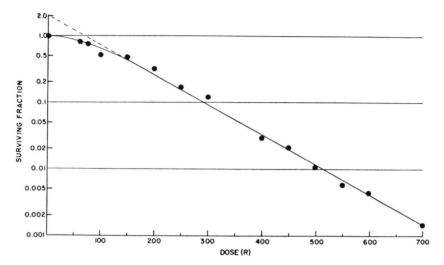

Fig. 6.8   Survival curve of human cervical tumour cells (HeLa cells), as a function of x-ray dose. The points fit the equation $F = 1 - (1 - e^{-D/96})^2$ within experimental uncertainty (Puck and Marcus, 1956)

From the previous argument, the probability of a single hit is given by

$$P_1 = 1 - e^{-kD}$$

The probability of n independent hits is then given by

$$P = (1 - e^{-kD})^n$$

If n hits are necessary to cause inactivation, the surviving fraction will be given by

$$\frac{N}{N_0} = 1 - (1 - e^{-kD})^n$$

The curve in Fig. 6.8 is of this form. At high doses $(kD \gg 1)$ this expression approaches

$$\frac{N}{N_0} = n e^{-kD}, \tag{6.3}$$

and if this exponential function be extrapolated back to $D = 0$, the line will intercept the ordinate at the point $N/N_0 = n$. Applying this procedure to the data in Fig. 6.8, we obtain the result $n = 2$ approximately. When this data is plotted on a linear scale we obtain a 'sigmoid' curve which is characteristic of survival doses for a wide variety of mammalian systems.

The fit between theory and the results of this experiment suggests that this 'multitarget' theory is valid in at least some circumstances. Clearly we are dealing here with a higher level of organisation than is found in viruses and bacteria, and additionally we see that the system is much more radiosensitive. In the data of Fig. 6.8 for example, the dose to reduce the surviving fraction to 37% is 200 rad, as distinct from 3×10^5 rad for the data on the potato virus illustrated in Fig. 6.7. Nevertheless we are still dealing with a situation in which the viability of each cell is independent of that of its neighbours. When we turn to more complex organisms such as small animals this independence is, of course, lost, and many new factors manifest themselves. Moreover, the variety of effects which may be used as indicators of biological damage becomes much greater.

Radiobiological studies at the cellular level of the type illustrated in Fig. 6.8 are concerned with damage to the mitotic function, to the extent that the reproductive capacity of the cell is lost, thereby preventing it from multiplying to form a visible colony. Other studies are concerned with the induction of genetic mutations.

When the effects of radiation on more complex organisms are being investigated, lethality of the radiation is an important aspect. It is found in radio-biological experiments on small animals that for doses less than a certain amount, the survival rate is virtually 100%. The data of Fig. 6.9 illustrate this point, and suggest that repair mechanisms can operate effectively at dose levels which, in rats irradiated with high energy (betatron-produced) x-rays, are in the region of 4–500 rads. The lethality is commonly expressed as the dose which would, on average, lead to a survival of 50% at a stated time after exposure, usually 30 days. This is denoted by the symbol $LD_{50/30}$. A few representative values are given in Table 6.3. For rats the $LD_{50/30}$ (for high-energy x- or γ-radiation) is in the

Table 6.3

$LD_{50(30)}$ values for total-body exposure of animals and other organisms to x- or γ-radiation (after Casarett, 1968)

	(rads)
Guinea-pig	400
Man	250–450
Mouse	550
Monkey	600
Rat	750
Song-sparrow	800
Goldfish	2300

region of 750 rads. Other important biological effects have been extensively investigated, for example the shortening of life-span in animals, the formation of cataracts of the lens of the eye, and the induction of leukaemia.

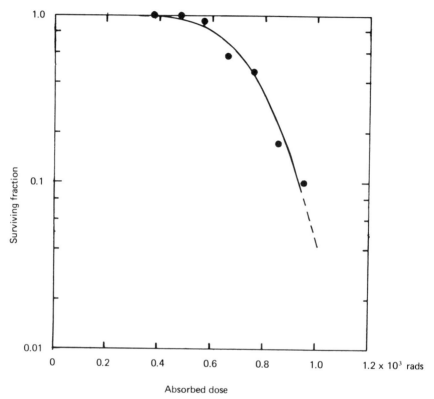

Fig. 6.9 Survival of rats following whole-body irradiation (from data of Fuller *et al.*, 1955)

Much practical interest centres on the possible use of radiobiological research to establish safe levels of radiation for radiation workers, and also for the public at large, exposed to environmental radiation from man-made sources, which represents an addition to the 'natural' background radiation from cosmic rays and natural environmental radioactivity. The principal problem is that it is very difficult to extrapolate, with any degree of reliability, to the very low levels of radiation which are relevant to the occupational or environmental situation. It is generally believed, however, that the permissible exposure is limited by the probability of deleterious genetic mutations and induction of cancers (including leukaemia) rather than other factors referred to in this section.

Much experience on the effects of x- and γ-radiation on human subjects has been gained from medical uses in radiotherapy and, to a more limited extent, in diagnostic radiology. In radiotherapy, accurately monitored doses of radiation, which may be substantial, are administered to carefully determined sites, in order to achieve regression, and ultimately the disappearance, of tumours.

These growths arise because of a local breakdown of the factors controlling tissue growth in the body. Unrestricted cell division then occurs. If the growth remains in the form of a 'self-contained' lesion it is termed a 'benign' tumour, and its effects will normally be limited to interference, by pressure or obstruction, with the function of neighbouring organs. Surgical intervention is normally necessary, and a cure is effected in a high proportion of cases. On the other hand, if the growth is invasive in nature, surgical procedures may not be practicable. Furthermore, fragments of the tissue may become detached and be transported to sites elsewhere in the body by means of the blood or the lymphatic systems, where they may act as centres for new growths termed **metastases**. It is in cases of these 'malignant' growths (whether metastatic or not) where radiation is often effective therapeutically. The exposure necessary to give the required radiation dose must be calculated carefully, and, in this connection, depth–dose curves of the type illustrated in Figs. 4.13 and 4.14 are made use of. Multiple field treatments are commonly used, to reduce the dose to the tissues overlying the tumour, and to the skin, and the use of megavoltage radiation is of great value in that it shows the phenomenon of 'build-up' to electronic equilibrium, referred to in connection with ionization dosimetry in section 3.5, which limits the surface dose to relatively low values.

Examples of radiation effects seen in connection with radiotherapeutic procedures are the reddening (or erythema) of the skin, which occurs when a skin dose of the order of 1000 rads of γ-radiation is given in the course of treatment. Loss of hair (epilation) from irradiated surfaces can also occur. Both these effects are temporary in normal radiotherapeutic practice. Responses affecting the whole system ('systemic effects') can also occur, although these are uncommon unless the radiation is being delivered internally by radioisotope administration. Such systemic effects include a reduction of the red-cell count, caused by irradiation of the red-cell-forming tissues in the bone marrow, and this effect may set a limit to the amount of ^{32}P which may be administered for the treatment of **polycythaemia** by radiation. Effects of this nature are often too complex to study quantitatively, either because of the qualitative nature of the effect being considered, or because of difficulties in calculating the absorbed dose to the tissues of interest. They are mentioned here to give the reader an introduction to the subject, which may be followed up in more detail in the references cited in the Further Reading at the end of this chapter.

We revert to the simpler effects observed at the cellular level, and now consider the effect of the LET in determining biological response. This involves taking a close interest in the microscopic distribution of energy within the biological material.

In the case of virus inactivation, high LET radiation is **less** effective, rad for rad, than that of low LET. The LET of the recoil protons from neutron irradiation extends over the range $20-100 \text{ keV} (\mu\text{m})^{-1}$, so that they deposit excessive energy in the virus whilst leaving much of the material, in effect, unirradiated. The same amount of absorbed dose, spread more uniformly throughout the virus preparation, would do more damage.

Conversely, if 2 or more 'hits' are required (as in the case of mitotic inhibition in mammalian cells), high LET radiation is often more effective, and we define the **Relative Biological Effectiveness**, (or RBE), which is the reciprocal of the ratio of absorbed doses necessary to produce the **same** degree of biological response in the two irradiations. Representative RBEs are given in Table 6.4, for several biological effects. More extensive studies have shown that in many situations, particularly in mammalian cells, RBEs for fast neutrons lie in the range 2-4. An example of a pair of survival curves, for γ-rays and fast neutrons, is given in Fig. 6.10.

Table 6.4 also illustrates that if a dose is given at a low dose-rate, or over a period of time, the biological effect is reduced, in the case of low-LET radiation. This is a consequence of the repair processes which can take place, to which

Table 6.4
RBEs for high and low LET radiations

Effect	Low LET		High LET	
	Single Exposure	Protracted Exposure	Single Exposure	Protracted Exposure
Life-shortening (Mouse)	1	0.2-0.4	1-5	4-8
Lense Opacification (Mouse)	1	0.3	2-9	2-9
(Man)	1	0.4		
Carcinogenisis (Mouse)	1	0.2-0.3	0.4-0.5	
Inactivation of Tobacco mosaic virus	1		0.86 (8.3 KeV x-rays†) 0.25 (1.5 KeV x-rays†)	
(Ra γ-rays = 1)			0.195 (4 MeV α-particles)	

After Spiers (1968).

† Not high LET in the accepted sense, but significantly higher than for Ra γ-rays.

reference has already been made. In the case of high LET radiation, the difference between a single and a protracted exposure is much less, suggesting that repair mechanisms are less effective.

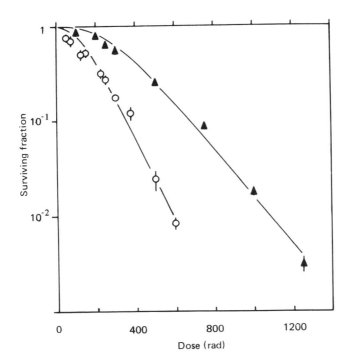

Fig. 6.10 Survival of Chinese hamster cells (measured as survival of cell reproductive capacity) following irradiation by γ-rays (▲) and 42 MeV d–Be neutrons (○) (Berry *et al.*, 1977)   (© 1977, American Roentgen Ray Society.)

For more detailed reading in this very extensive field of study, the reader is referred to texts by Casarett (1968) and Alper (1979) listed at the end of this chapter.

6.3.1 The role of oxygen

At the molecular level, it is generally considered that radiation damage is caused, in part at least, by oxidation processes which are aided by products, such as hydroxyl ions, of the radiolysis of the water in which cellular material is normally bathed. It is to be expected therefore, that the radiosensitivity of biological material will be affected by the presence of dissolved oxygen, and that radiosensitivity will in fact increase as the partial pressure of dissolved oxygen ('oxygen tension') is increased. This is found to be the case, and is known as the 'oxygen effect'.

This phenomenon has important practical consequences. For example, certain regions of tumours are sometimes very poorly supplied with blood, and it follows that these will be regions where the oxygen used up by metabolic processes will not be replaced at an adequate rate. The oxygen tension will therefore be low, and these regions of tumour will be radioresistant. It is widely held that the failure of some tumours to respond to radiation treatment may be due to the increased radioresistivity of poorly-oxygenated cells. One consequence of this has been the development of 'hyperbaric oxygen therapy', in which the patient is placed in an atmosphere of oxygen, at a pressure of 3 atmospheres. The increased radiosensitivity of the poorly-oxygenated tumour cells greatly exceeds the small increase in radiosensitivity of the normal, well-oxygenated tissues. Tumours which are normally radioresistant become radiosensitive, and some limited success has been reported in the treatment of lung cancer by this method. The increase of radiosensitivity may be quantitated in terms of the reciprocal of the ratio of doses necessary to produce a given biological effect, and the **Oxygen Enhancement Ratio** is defined in this way. Ratios of 2.5–3 for well-oxygenated to poorly-oxygenated tissues are typical of experimental studies in this field.

In the case of high LET radiation, damage by locally-produced OH (and possibly other oxidising radicals) is relatively large, and the added effect of dissolved oxygen in tissue fluids is not so marked. Oxygen enhancement ratios in the case of irradiation by high LET radiation are not so great (~2), and so the poorly-oxygenated regions of tumours are not at such a disadvantage in therapeutic irradiation. Therapy by means of fast neutrons is becoming established as an advantageous method for poorly-oxygenated tumours, after a long period of research and clinical trial (see, for example, the detailed study by Catterall and Bewley, 1979), and centres for the development of neutron therapy are becoming more numerous. Cyclotrons are in use for this work, and (to give a typical example) the (d,n) reaction on beryllium using 15 MeV deuterons, as described in section 6.2, is used to produce a suitable fast neutron beam. Low voltage accelerators, using the DT reaction which produces 14 MeV neutrons, are also in use for this work. A difficulty with both these methods is that the penetration of the beam is not entirely adequate for deep-seated tumours. It is likely that cyclotrons of somewhat higher energy will be built to produce neutron beams of greater penetration for future work.

An alternative approach is to introduce small 'seeds' of neutron-emitting isotopes into the tumour mass. Californium-252 decaying by spontaneous fission is undergoing trials for this purpose. The relatively low penetration of fission neutrons (which have a spectrum peaking at about 1 MeV) is not a disadvantage in this mode of administering the radiation dose.

Although higher energy neutrons are needed if the beam penetration is to be substantially better than that of 250 kV x-rays, it should be noted that the LET of the faster recoiling protons will be somewhat lower than those resulting from

15 MeV deuterons on beryllium. The benefits of the neutrons may therefore become less marked as the energy is increased. But to offset this there is the consideration that the neutrons may themselves induce spallation and other nuclear reactions at the point where the neutron is absorbed. The products of these reactions will often have a high LET, and consequently a high RBE, and an oxygen enhancement ratio which is sufficiently low for the potential benefits of neutron therapy to be fully achieved in practice.

6.4 NEUTRON DETECTION AND DOSIMETRY

Neutrons carry no electric charge, and are therefore unable to ionize matter directly. In order to detect neutrons, therefore, it is necessary to detect charged particles set in motion by elastic collisions or nuclear reactions. A second group of methods is based on the production of induced radioactivity in suitable detecting materials (for example foils or pellets). We shall refer briefly to the principles used in neutron detection and dosimetry, but without including a great deal of technical detail, for which the reader is referred to specialised texts.

6.4.1 Detectors based on elastic scattering

We have seen (section 6.1) that nuclei struck by a fast neutron recoil with energies up to a value given by

$$E' = E \left(\frac{A-1}{A+1} \right)^2 \tag{6.4}$$

Light nuclei therefore take up a substantial fraction of the energy and, in the limiting case of a head-on collision with protons, the whole of the kinetic energy may be transferred. Hydrogenous materials are therefore used extensively in neutron detection. Proportional counters with a hydrogen filling are found useful for neutrons with energies above about 200 keV, and can give a good degree of discrimination against γ-radiation.

The spectrum of proton recoils from monoenergetic neutron collisions is flat, extending down to $E = 0$ (Fig. 6.11). It follows, in principle at least, that the proton recoil spectrum can be 'unfolded' to give the spectrum of incident neutrons. In practice the shape of the proton recoil spectrum is modified by the 'wall effect' (see below) but this can be allowed for in the unfolding procedure.

The range of protons in hydrogen at atmospheric pressure is sufficiently large to make desirable a counter of somewhat large dimensions. It is advantageous to fill the counter to a pressure of a few atmospheres, or to mix a heavy noble gas (for example krypton) with the hydrogen to reduce this range. In normal circumstances, a proportion of the recoiling protons will strike the walls of the chamber, and this effect will result in the production of pulses of reduced height.

As an alternative to a purely gaseous filling, a solid hydrogenous material (for example paraffin wax) may be introduced into the chamber to act as a 'radiator' for protons which are then detected by the counter gas. This increases the detection efficiency and by suitable design can reduce the wall effect.

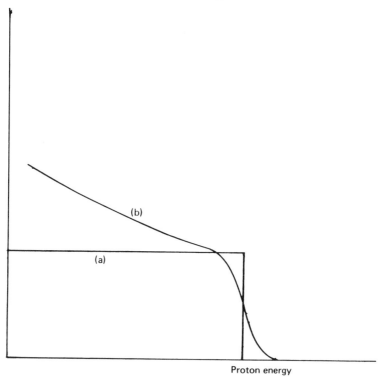

Fig. 6.11 Proton recoil spectrum from monoenergetic neutrons (a) disregarding the wall effect (b) including the wall effect and the effect of finite energy resolution

Scintillation counters have been developed for fast neutrons. A plastic scintillator will readily detect neutrons, but the efficiency for gamma radiation is appreciable and difficulty is experienced in discriminating against this. A special scintillator, consisting of zinc sulphide mixed with plastic material, is in wide use, known as a Hornyak 'button'. The recoil protons produced in the plastic are detected, with high efficiency and light output, by the zinc sulphide. Discrimination against γ-radiation is practicable for neutrons with energies in excess of about 5 MeV.

6.4.2 Use of nuclear reactions

Certain nuclear reactions are extensively used for slow neutron detection. The $^{10}B(n,\alpha)^7Li$ is the best-known example. If a counter is filled with boron in suitable gaseous form (boron trifluoride being widely used for this purpose), it may be operated in the proportional region, and will detect slow neutrons with good efficiency. The reaction is exoergic by 2.78 MeV, and although 94% of the lithium nuclei are produced in an excited state (at 480 keV) above the ground state) an energy of 2.3 MeV is available as kinetic energy of the recoiling α-particles and ^{7}Li nuclei, to produce a strong pulse, enabling good discrimination against γ-radiation to be achieved. Such counters are also used for the detection of fast neutrons, if surrounded by a few cm of moderating material (polythene, paraffin wax) and approximate measurements of absolute fluxes are possible by this method.

An ionization chamber filled with boron trifluoride is an efficient detector for slow neutrons and, if suitably large, can be made sensitive to the low fluxes which are relevant in the field of radiation protection. Boron can be used to 'load' scintillator material to produce a scintillation counter sensitive to slow neutrons. For the detection of very small neutron fluxes, a photographic emulsion loaded with boron-containing compounds is an extremely sensitive detector. It may be exposed to the neutron flux for long periods (several weeks if necessary) and then developed. The tracks caused by the α-particles are readily observed in the optical microscope, and may be counted to yield quantative results.

Fission counters are in widespread use for the detection of slow and fast neutrons. The fissile material is introduced into an ionization chamber or proportional counter, and the choice of fissile material is determined by the use to which the device is to be put. ^{235}U is fissionable by slow and fast neutrons, ^{238}U by fast neutrons ($>$1.5 MeV) only, and ^{237}Np is also available for fast neutron detectors (fission threshold 0.6 MeV). The proportional counter yields very large pulses ($\sim$180 MeV) so discrimination against α-radiation and large fluxes of γ-radiation is possible.

6.4.3 Pulse shape discrimination

The ability of a scintillation counter to discriminate against γ-radiation can be greatly improved by making use of the differing luminescent decay characteristics for different radiations. In the case of organic materials, two components of light output are observed. In the case of anthracene, for example, the 'slow' and 'fast' components have luminescent decay times of 370 and 33 ns respectively. It is observed that the slow component is more strongly excited by high LET particles than by electrons or γ-rays. The shape of the pulses from the two radiation types are therefore sufficiently different for discrimination by electronic methods to be possible. This is achieved by integration followed by double differentiation of the signal. The time of zero crossing of the doubly differentiated pulse depends on the strength of the slow component, being **later** the stronger the **slow** component of the pulses. The pulses which are passed to the scaler or multi-channel analyser can be selected on the basis of their zero crossing time, and enhanced discrimination against γ-rays thereby achieved.

Because the strength of the slow component depends also on the energy of the high-LET particles, the system can be adapted to provide information on the spectral distribution of the neutrons. Although it is not the intention here to discuss methods of neutron spectroscopy, this extension of a basic detection method is mentioned as an example of a relatively simple method of obtaining information on the energy distribution of a neutron flux.

6.4.4 Threshold detectors

From time to time it is useful to measure neutron fluxes by means of the radio-activity induced in a small sample of material in foil or powdered form. This method facilitates the measurement of the spatial distribution of neutrons around a source, or the distribution in an extended medium, as the samples to be activated need be no more than a few mm in size. The measurement of an integrated flux is possible, although the duration of the irradiation must be short compared with the half-life of the activity produced, if a true measurement of fluence (integral of flux with respect to time) is to be obtained.

If reactions are chosen which have a definite threshold, this method will measure only those neutrons in excess of this threshold energy, although the relative sensitivity at different energies will be dependent upon the way in which the cross-section will vary with energy. A threshold detector is small and portable, and can normally be measured with a Geiger counter, if the product nucleus is a β- or γ-emitter. Examples of such detectors are $^{32}S(n,p)^{32}P$ and $^{27}Al(n, \alpha)^{24}Na$, with effective thresholds at 3 MeV and 8 MeV respectively. The sulphur is normally fabricated in small pellets of elemental sulphur, and the aluminium is most conveniently used as foil or thin sheet. Many substances are activated by thermal neutrons, and the choice of detector is determined by the need for a reasonably high activation cross-section and a half-life in a suitable range. This must be sufficiently long to be capable of integrating the flux over the required period without approaching the equilibrium expressed in (2.6). If the half-life is unnecessarily long, however, the disintegration rate during the subsequent counting period will be inconveniently low.

For thermal neutrons indium foils are often used, in which the activity produced by the $^{115}In(n,\gamma)^{116}In$ reaction has a half-life of 54 minutes. Indium has a high capture cross-section ($\sigma_{thermal} = 200$ barn) for all neutron energies below 1.4 eV, peaking to a strong resonance at this energy.

6.4.5 Neutron Dosimetry

It is practicable to design small ionization chambers using the Bragg-Gray principle (section 3.5) in order to determine the absorbed dose in a suitable wall material. Such a material may be, for example, a plastic of known composition to obtain a relatively simple atomic composition, or may be a more complex mixture designed to achieve tissue equivalence over the range of neutron energies for which it will be used. As an example of the former approach, a 'CH' plastic (for example polystyrene, or a mixture of polystyrene, polythene and graphite) is used, or a 'CH$_2$' plastic (that is polythene). For tissue equivalence, it is desirable to include some nitrogenous material (for instance in the form of nylon), and small amounts of silicon and calcium. Detailed formulations for such mixtures are given in the literature (see Holm and Berry, 1970).

Because the protons and recoiling nuclei associated with neutron absorption have a much shorter range than electrons of comparable energy, it is not easy to satisfy the Bragg–Gray criterion of small size. It is therefore desirable to design chambers so that they are homogeneous, and this involves producing a filling gas which has the same stopping power, and also the same neutron absorption characteristics, as the walls. This presents no problems in the case of a 'CH' or 'CH$_2$' chamber (for which acetylene and ethylene respectively may be used) but is more difficult in the case of chambers which are intended to be tissue equivalent. A gas mixture of 32.4% carbon dioxide, 64.4% methane and 3.2% nitrogen has been described and used for this purpose.

Another difficulty in designing a chamber for fast neutrons is that saturation is more difficult to achieve, because of the very dense nature of the ionization caused by the proton and other recoils. Correction may have to be applied for this.

A third problem concerns the correction of neutron dosimeter readings for the presence of γ-rays. This may be carried out by pairing the neutron chamber with one which is relatively insensitive to neutrons (that is, graphite walls and CO$_2$ filling), but a rather simpler method is to use photographic film as a γ-ray monitor. A third method uses thermoluminescence as the dosimetric principle (see section 3.5), when different isotopes of the same element (for example ^{6}Li or ^{7}Li) may be incorporated into thermoluminescent material (for instance LiF) to utilise their different properties: ^{6}LiF has a moderately high response because of the occurence of the ^{6}Li$(n, \alpha)^3$H reaction, whereas ^{7}LiF is relatively insensitive to neutrons.

Neutron dosimetry may thus be carried out on a sound basis, with an accuracy only slightly inferior to that achievable with γ-rays or x-rays.

6.5 NEUTRON ACTIVATION ANALYSIS

The production of radioactive isotopes by neutron irradiation can be applied to the analysis of small quantities of material — an irradiation with thermal neutrons (usually in a reactor) is followed by gamma-spectroscopy to identify the radio-isotopes present and to determine their amounts. Usually specific elements are being looked for on the basis of known γ-ray lines; and a sample of known mass is usually irradiated in the same flux to provide a calibration spectrum. The sensitivity of the method varies greatly from one element to another depending upon the cross-section of the (n, γ) reaction and the intensity of the strongest

γ-lines, which, in turn, is determined by the decay rate of the product and the details of its decay scheme.

The samples to be irradiated are placed in an aluminium container and can be irradiated in a reactor facility for a few weeks. After irradiation the material can be removed from the container and examined by scintillation counter or Ge(Li) detector; but the spectrum will often be swamped by the relatively large amount of activity produced from sodium (invariably present in biological material) and so some form of radiochemical separation may need to be carried out.

Elements of potential biological interest which can be detected down to a few nanograms include antimony, arsenic, iodine and copper. The technique is well-established in biological research although of course is not confined to this field.

Perhaps more relevant to medical applications of nuclear physics is the technique of *in vivo* neutron activation analysis which is currently used in an increasing number of laboratories throughout the world. In this application of neutron physics the human subject, or patient, can be given a small dose of fast neutrons which, when moderated in the body, will undergo capture by a variety of elements, and will, in some instances, yield products which are radioactive. These can be measured by a suitable assemblage of γ-ray detectors, usually by placing the subject in a 'whole-body' counter, which is a heavily shielded chamber of sufficient size to accommodate the patient (usually on a couch) with several detectors positioned so that the system as a whole possesses a reasonably uniform response to radiation from all parts of the body. Several elements may be studied by this method. Sodium in the body is activated to ^{24}Na (15 hr half-life) and the first proposals for the study of *in vivo* neutron activation analysis stemmed from the realisation that the measurement of ^{24}Na would be a good monitor following an accidental exposure to fast neutrons. Clinical applications have been mainly in connection with other elements. The measurement of total body calcium is an example of the clinical use of the technique. This can be carried out by using the ^{48}Ca(n,γ)^{49}Ca reaction, even though ^{48}Ca is present in ordinary calcium only to the extent of about 0.2%. In certain pathological conditions, some of the calcium in the skeleton (which normally accounts for more than 99% of the calcium in the body) is resorbed into the blood, and the subsequent loss of calcium from the body calls for chemotherapy. This is the condition known as **osteoporosis**. A measurement of total-body calcium, repeated at intervals, can give an indication of the response of the patient to treatment. A further example is the measurement of copper in the body. In the hereditary condition known as Wilson's disease, mechanisms for copper metabolism break down, and abnormally large concentrations develop in the liver. The same is true to a lesser extent in primary biliary cirrhosis. The amounts of copper (and hence, knowing the approximate liver mass, the copper **concentrations**) can be determined by using the ^{63}Cu(n,γ)^{64}Cu reaction and then measuring the activity of the 12 hr β^+ activity of ^{64}Cu. By the design of suitable neutral collimators, the beam can be confined to the region of the liver, thereby keeping the total body irradiation down to as low a value as possible.

As an alternative to the measurement of induced radioactivity, use can be made of the 'prompt' γ-radiation emitted in radiative capture. This has a spectrum which is characteristic of the product nucleus, and can be used for identification and determination of the mass present. In this case the product nucleus need not, of course, be radioactive. This method is used for the measurement of nitrogen in the body, using the 10.8 MeV γ-ray emitted in the ^{14}N(n,γ) reaction. The amount of nitrogen in the body is an index of total body protein, and the technique is of value in all cases where nitrogen balance studies are needed, for example in postoperative dietary therapy. Because of the strong background of γ-radiation from the neutron-producing reaction in the cyclotron (for example the 10 MeV proton bombardment of a lithium target), it is usual to use a pulsed beam technique in which the counting system is gated 'off' during the pulse and the subsequent slowing-down time of the neutron, and is brought 'on' during the period of neutron capture.

As a final example of analysis by 'prompt-gamma' radiation, the study of cadmium may be mentioned. Because of the very high capture cross-section of ^{114}Cd for thermal neutrons, the method can be used for very low concentrations of cadmium. This is important in view of the role of cadmium as a potentially toxic element in the environment. The industrial uses of cadmium also suggest a potential occupational hazard. This technique (using either a pulsed cyclotron source or a sealed α-beryllium source of neutrons) is used to detect and measure the elevated cadmium levels found in cadmium workers, and concentrations in the liver down to a few parts per million can be measured. Levels in the kidneys (where it is thought that the risk of toxicity is greatest) can also be measured in some circumstances. For further details of this interesting area of applied neutron physics the reader may consult original papers, for example Spinks (1979), Harvey *et al.* (1973) and Vartsky *et al.* (1977) for work on calcium, nitrogen and cadmium respectively.

FURTHER READING

Alper, T. (1979) *Cellular Radiobiology* Cambridge
Casarett, A. P. (1968) *Radiation Biology* Prentice-Hall
Catterall, M. and Bewley, D. K. (1979) *Fast neutrons in the treatment of cancer* Academic Press

REFERENCES

Berry, R. J., Bance, D. A., Barnes, D. W. H., Cox, R., Goodhead, D. T., Sansom, J. M. and Thacker, J. (1977) *Amer. J. Roentgenol.,* **129**, 717

Burch, P. R. J. (1957a) *Radiation Res., 6*, 289

Burch, P. R. J. (1957b) *Brit. Journ. Radiol., 30*, 524

Fuller, J. B., Chen, I., Laughlin, J. S. and Harvey, R. A. (1955) *Radiation Res., 3*, 423

Goodhead, D. T., Berry, R. J., Bance, D. A., Gray, P. and Stedeford, J. B. H. (1977) *Amer. J. Roentgenol.* **129**, 709

Hannan, W. J., Porter, D., Lawson, R. C. and Railton, R. (1973) *Phys. Med. Biol.,* **18**, 808

Harvey, T. C., Dykes, P. W., Chen, N. S., Ettinger, K. V., Jain, S., James, H., Chettle, D. R., Fremlin, J. H. and Thomas, B. (1973) *Lancet,* **II**, 395

Holm, N. W. and Berry, R. J. (eds.) (1970). See Further Reading for Chapter 3.

ICRP/ICRU Report of the RBE committee (1963) *Health Phys.* **9**, 357

Lea, D. E. (1955) *Actions of radiation on living cells* Cambridge

Puck, T. T. and Marcus, P. I. (1956) *J. Expt. Med.,* **103**, 653

Spiers, F. W. (1968). See Further Reading for Chapter 5

Spinks, T. J. (1979) *Phys. Med. Biol.,* **24**, 976

The Radiochemical Manual (1966). See Further Reading for Chapter 2

Vartsky, D., Ellis, K. J., Chen, N. S. and Cohn, S. H. (1977) *Phys. Med. Biol.,* **22**, 1085

Walker, J. (1967) *Rep. Prog. Phys., 30*, 285

Watt, B. E. (1952) *Phys. Rev.,* **87**, 1037

CHAPTER 7

Other accelerator-based applications in medicine and biology

7.1 *X*-RAYS INDUCED BY PROTONS AND OTHER HEAVY PARTICLES, FOR ANALYSIS

The production of characteristic *x*-rays by electron bombardment is a familiar process, as is its interpretation in terms of the differences in energy levels of the singly-ionized atom. Characteristic *x*-rays also provide the basis for several techniques of elemental analysis, that is, analysis in terms of elements present. One such technique has led to the production and widespread use of the electron microprobe, in which a demagnified electron beam is allowed to impinge on the sample to be analysed, and is scanned across it. The emitted *x*-rays are detected by a proportional counter or solid-state (Si(Li)) detector, and the output converted to a signal for display on a video system. If the electronics includes a pulse-height analyser adjusted to accept the characteristic *x*-rays from one element, the display will show the concentration of that element alone, and can be subjected to quantitative interpretation. Another technique makes use of *x*-ray fluorescence, by irradiating the sample with an intense beam of a continuous *x*-ray spectrum and by analysis of the fluorescent radiation using a curved crystal spectrometer or solid-state detector. This is not a scanning system but is capable of detecting considerably lower levels of concentration.

The electron microprobe can produce an electron beam 1 μm in diameter without difficulty, and, bearing in mind that the penetration of 20–40 keV electrons in typical specimens will be of the order of 1–2 μm only, it will be seen that analysis can be carried out on volume elements of the order of 10^{-12} (cm)^3 only. Concentrations down to about 50–100 parts per million (ppm) of an element can be detected, in favourable circumstances. In *x*-ray fluorescence analysis, the lower limit of detection is as low as 1–2 ppm, but several grams of material are required for optimum performance.

Against this background we may now discuss briefly the use of 'nuclear' particles (protons, α-particles, and heavy ions) for elemental analysis of biological material.

When matter is bombarded by protons, the beam loses energy by the ionization processes which we analysed in Chapter 1. Occasionally ionization from an inner shell occurs, followed by characteristic x-ray emission. If ionization occurs in the K shell, the x-ray spectrum is the same as that observed in electron bombardment and in fluorescence. However, if L shell ionization occurs, the ionization probability of the three subshells will not, in general, be the same as in conventional methods of ionization, so the relative intensity of the lines from different subshells may be different.

The amount of bremsstrahlung produced by proton bombardment is much less than that observed in electron bombardment, essentially because of the much greater mass of the proton. We discuss this later in this section, but should point out here that the low bremsstrahlung yield greatly improves the peak-to-background ratio in the spectra, enabling much lower levels of concentration to be detected than is the case in the electron microprobe. Therein lies the interest and importance of proton-induced x-rays, in the present context.

The cross-section, σ, for inner-shell ionization has been investigated extensively in recent years. It rises rapidly with proton energy, reaching a broad maximum when the proton velocity is of the same order as the Bohr orbital velocity appropriate to the shell being ionized. That is, the maximum cross-section occurs when

$$v_p = \alpha Z c, \tag{7.1}$$

or when

$$E_p = \tfrac{1}{2} M_p c^2 (\alpha Z_{\text{eff}})^2 \quad \text{or} \quad \frac{M_p}{m} E_k. \tag{7.2}$$

In these expressions, α is the fine structure constant,[†] M_p and m are the proton and electron masses respectively, and Z_{eff} (in the classical treatment of the Bohr–Sommerfeld atom) is the effective atomic number, taking into account the screening effect of the orbital electrons.[‡] v_p and E_p are respectively the velocity and energy of the protons.

We see that to achieve maximum cross-section, relatively high values of proton energy are needed; for the K shell of iron, for example, $E_k = 7.11$ keV, and (7.2) points to a proton energy of several MeV. However, at substantially lower energies, the yield of x-rays is still considerable, and much work has been

---

† $\alpha = e^2/\hbar c$, or, in the form suitable for use with S.I. units, $\mu_0 c e^2/2h$. In each form its numerical value is $(137.04)^{-1}$.

‡ More accurately, Z_{eff} takes into account the screening of the **inner** electronic charge, but not the outer screening. The latter further reduces E_k to a value which is less than $\tfrac{1}{2} m c^2 (\alpha Z_{\text{eff}})^2$ by a factor θ, known as a **screening number**. We may overlook this distinction here, as we are not pursuing the theoretical treatment of inner-shell ionization; but for a detailed analysis of this, the reader may consult the paper by Merzbacher and Lewis (1958) and the review by Garcia *et al.* (1973).

carried out at energies of a few hundred keV only. For elemental analysis, the optimum energy appears to be 2–3 MeV.

The quantity σE_k^2 has been found to be approximately the same function of E_p/E_k for all elements, and so the data for different elements may be displayed on a single curve. This is illustrated in Fig. 7.1, from which it may also be seen that, when $E_p \ll \dfrac{M_p}{m} E_k$, the cross-section is proportional approximately to the fourth power of the proton energy. This is consistent with theoretical treatments at low energies. The quantity E_p/E_k is frequently termed the excitation ratio, and is denoted by U.

The data of Fig. 7.1 implies a very strong inverse Z dependence, especially at low proton energies. For if

$$\sigma E_k^2 = \text{const.} \left(\frac{E_p}{E_k} \right)^4 \tag{7.3}$$

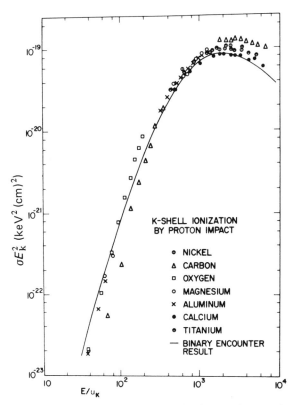

Fig. 7.1 Inner-shell ionization by proton-bombardment. The quantity σE_k^2 is the same function of E_p/E_k for all the elements investigated (Garcia, 1971)

and if $E_k \propto Z_{eff}^2$ approximately, it follows that we might expect the cross-section at a fixed proton energy to vary as Z^{-12} approximately. Experimentally the dependence is not so strong, but a variation of Z^{-8} or Z^{-9} is observed (Fig. 7.2) pointing to the importance of having a relatively high proton energy available, if it is desired to excite the K shell of high-Z elements.

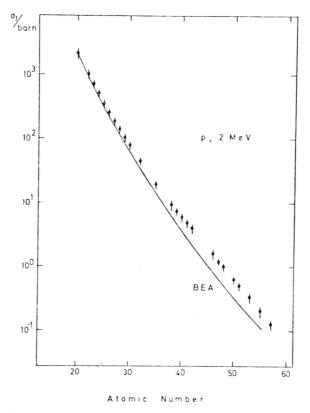

Fig. 7.2 K-shell ionization cross-section plotted as a function of target atomic number (proton bombardment energy 2 MeV) (Raith *et al.* 1977)

The yield from thick targets has also been examined experimentally. A rapid rise with increasing proton energy ($\propto E_p^4$ or E_p^5) is observed, and also the strong inverse dependence on atomic number already noted.

The yield of L x-rays is substantial. Again the parameter $U(= E_p/E_L)$ is a useful guide to the expected thick target yield. For heavy elements, analysis by particle-induced x-ray emission is usually based on observations of L x-rays.

Accelerators used for proton-induced x-ray analysis are usually Cockcroft-Walton machines or small van de Graaff accelerators. They will usually be fitted with a multi-way target chamber, with remote-controlled target changing, and the *x*-ray detector is normally a lithium-drifted silicon detector. One of the principal advantages of this method of analysis is that several elements may be looked for simultaneously, and so it is usual to route the detector output signal to a multichannel analyser which may be connected 'on-line' to a computer for analysis of the spectrum and comparison with standards. A method of beam current monitoring and integration is also needed. The current will normally need to be limited to 20–30 nA for biological work, to avoid degradation of the sample and consequent changes in concentration, due to loss of volatile components.

For the preparation of thin samples, the material must be prepared in solution or in suspension, and may then be deposited by means of a 'nebuliser' on to a suitable backing foil, which may be a thin layer of organic material such as 'formvar' (as used for the mounting of specimens for electron microscopy), with possibly an added evaporated layer of aluminium to prevent charging effects in the beam. A **thick** target will normally require to be several tens of micrometres thick, and may be in the form of a compressed pellet (of, for example, freeze-dried material) or a section cut by microtome, or a polished metallic or mineralogical specimen. The development of methods of specimen preparation is of central importance, and each type of specimen may call for the development of particular preparation techniques appropriate to the material being handled. If a 'thin target technique' is being used, it is necessary to deposit a **known mass** of material on to the backing material, or to deposit the material from a known volume of suspension. The *x*-ray output will be proportional to the mass of material, and the information obtained will be in terms of a known mass of material. Thin target techniques are very suitable for the determination of small amounts of material dissolved in water, for the study of organic material which has been digested into aqueous solution, or for study of the composition of samples of dust deposited on to filters through which a known volume of air has passed in the course of specimen collection. Thick targets yield information directly in terms of **concentration** rather than mass, and so this information is of value in a wide variety of biological materials, for example the determination of the concentrations of trace elements or minor elements in biological tissue from organs such as the kidney or liver. A thick target may be a polished metallurgical or mineralogical sample. The information from a thick target will often require correcting for self-absorption of *x*-radiation leaving the target, usually from the same side as the incident proton beam, and in this connection it will be noted that this correction may rise rather rapidly with proton energy, due to increased penetration of the protons into the sample. This is proportional to $E^{3/2}$ or E^2, at the energies of interest to us. The rapid rise of the absorption correction with energy is an important reason for limiting the energy of the protons to a value not more than 3 or 4 MeV. This is particularly important if the L spectrum is being used for the study of heavy elements, where the absorption correction can be quite high even at proton energies below 1 MeV.

A further correction is needed for the differing stopping powers of the materials being examined. This will normally be important when comparing a specimen of, say, organic material with a pure sample of the element of interest. The nature of the correction may be understood by noting that the removal of the bulk of the material comprising a standard, and its replacement with an equal mass of material of lower atomic number, would **reduce** the range of the protons (v. section 1.3); hence, the determination of trace metal concentration in an organic material would need a **positive** correction to allow for this. It is normally much more satisfactory to make standards of known amounts of material, distributed throughout a 'matrix', with an atomic composition rather similar to that of the material being investigated. Calibration samples of elements dispersed in blood or gelatine are very suitable for work with biological material.

From thin targets, the concentration can, of course, be determined, if the mass of material, as well as the absolute intensity of the x-rays is known, together with cross-section measurements or measurements on samples which themselves are of known mass. This indirect method may be of value in some circumstances. A detailed investigation of the preparation of biological tissue samples has been given by Kemp *et al.* (1975).

It should be pointed out that material being prepared for analysis will normally require to be desiccated. A determination of concentration will then usually require to be corrected by a factor equal to the fraction by weight of water normally present in 'wet' samples of that tissue.

An advance was made when it was realised that a sample can be bombarded in air, if the proton beam is allowed to leave the machine through a thin foil. Specimen preparation techniques can then be relaxed considerably, because the sample does not have to be introduced into the vacuum system of the accelerator. Furthermore, there is no need to apply an evaporated gold or aluminium layer to the surface because surface charging and discharging effects are absent in air. There is also much less risk of loss of volatile material from the sample. An example of this technique is described by Huda and Bewley (1979).

Applications of proton-induced x-ray analysis have extended into many fields. Only a few can be mentioned here. In environmental studies, samples of water can be analysed by evaporating a few drops on to a plastic substrate, or by floating a graphite foil into the water sample. An example is illustrated in Fig. 7.3, in which the measurements are calibrated by means of an added element not expected to be normally present in the sample. Other environmental samples can be prepared from filters through which air has been drawn. If the deposit is formed on a strip of filter paper moving slowly across the air current, the strip can be subsequently scanned to give the variation with time of the amount of material deposited. This can be of value in environmental studies, for example, in correlating atmospheric pollution with meteorological conditions or with the atmospheric discharge of effluent from factories. These targets are examples of 'thin' targets, as defined earlier.

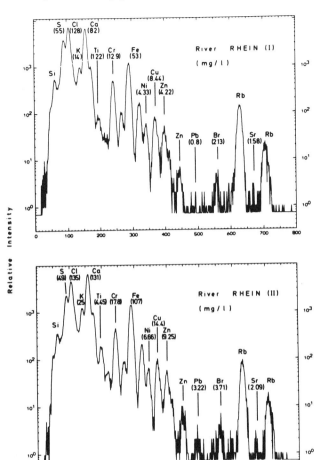

Fig. 7.3 Proton-induced *x*-ray spectra of river water (a) upstream and (b) downstream with respect to a chemical processing factory. The concentrations of several elements are shown in parentheses on the spectra, expressed in parts per million
(Raith *et al.* 1977)

In the field of pathology, studies of liver and kidney tissue obtained post mortem from human subjects have been reported (Dyson *et al.* 1978). It has been known for some time (for example Hunt *et al.* 1963) that certain disease states may be correlated with abnormalities in the concentration of minor elements in these tissues. In cirrhosis of the liver, for example, the metabolism of copper is interfered with, and the element accumulates in the liver, producing concentrations which are considerably elevated above normal (Fig. 7.4). The

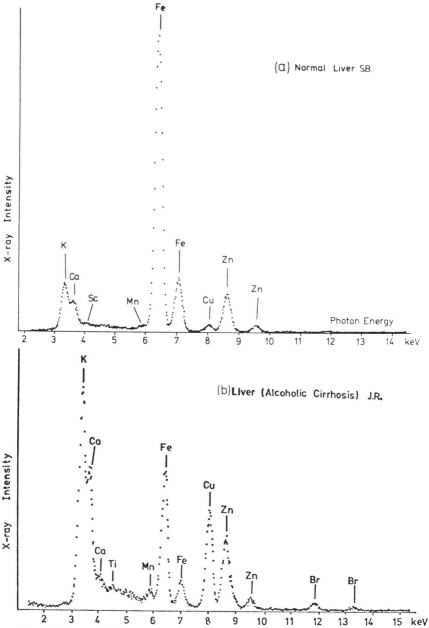

Fig. 7.4 Proton-induced x-ray spectra of liver samples obtained post mortem (a) from tissue believed to be normal, and (b) from a case of alcoholic cirrhosis. In the latter case, analysis of the data showed that the copper level was substantially higher than in the normal liver (60 ppm as compared with 9.5 ppm). The iron was much diminished (50 ppm as compared with 429 ppm), and this effect was associated with clinical anaemia (Dyson et al. 1978)

concentration of zinc may also be changed. For this type of work, thick targets have been used, prepared by sectioning and freeze-drying. Calibration may be achieved by adding known concentrations of these elements to a convenient matrix, for example blood.

The **sensitivity** for an element is defined as dN/da, where N is the counting rate per unit beam current in a given geometry and a the amount of the element in the target. It depends upon a number of factors, the most important of which is the ionization cross-section for the element in question. If we take, as a starting point for discussion, an element with Z in the region of 20, the counting rate for K radiation, in a given geometry, will fall rapidly as Z is increased, because of the strong inverse Z dependence of cross-section. The sensitivity therefore falls with increasing Z, until the point is reached at which the L spectrum is able to dominate the photon flux reaching the detector. The sensitivity again becomes high for this region of atomic number. Fig. 7.5 illustrates that the choice of the

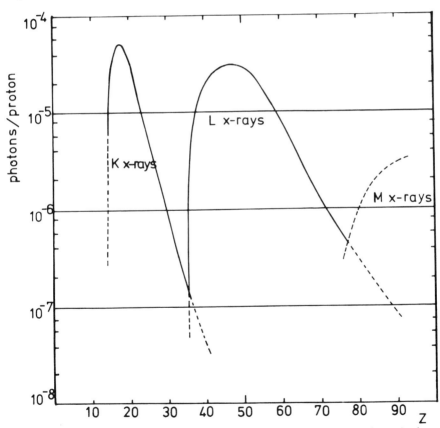

Fig. 7.5 Sensitivity of a system for proton-induced *x*-ray analysis, as determined by the counting rate per unit current for different atomic numbers of target material (Dyson, 1975)

spectrum to be used for analysis therefore depends on the atomic number of the element of interest.

If the energy of the bombarding protons is increased, the sensitivity (as just defined) will normally increase. However, in the case of low or medium-Z elements, the maximum cross-section, as we have seen from Fig. 7.1, is reached for proton energies of a few MeV. A further factor to be considered in this connection is the amount of self-absorption experienced by the emerging radiation, if the radiation is observed from the incident surface.

The other quantity of importance is the lower limit of detection. This depends upon the level of the continuum background, in addition to the considerations mentioned above. The bremsstrahlung consists of two main components – the **primary** bremsstrahlung from the proton beam, and the **secondary** bremsstrahlung, from 'knocked-on' electrons. Fig. 7.6 illustrates that the latter component is much the stronger of the two at low photon energies, and it is this factor which sets a lower limit to the concentration of elements which may be detected from

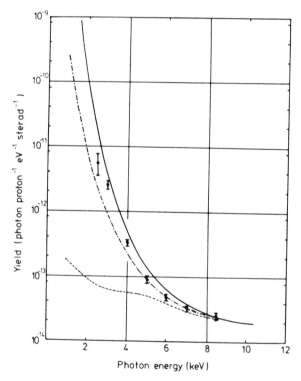

Fig. 7.6 The bremsstrahlung continuum obtained by bombardment of an aluminium target with 480 keV protons. Φ Experimental observations; - - - - - - - calculated primary proton bremsstrahlung; — · — · — primary bremsstrahlung plus the effect of electrons ejected from the K-shell; ——————— primary bremsstrahlung plus the effect of **all** s electrons ejected by proton collisions (Ward and Dyson, 1978)

a thick target. If the photon energy at the bremsstrahlung maximum is well below the characteristic radiation energy, the lower limit of detection will improve (fall) gradually as the proton energy is increased, because of the rise in ionization cross-section. But if the energy is increased beyond a certain limit (or if the characteristic radiation lies in an unfavourable part of the continuum), the background spectrum will encroach on the relevant energy channels, and the concentration at the lower limit of detection will increase. Fig. 7.7 illustrates the progressive change of the background continuum as the proton energy is increased.

Yet a further factor to be taken into account as the proton energy is increased is the onset of nuclear reactions in the light elements in the organic matrix. This will contribute to the γ-ray background at the detector, which will inevitably cause some increase in the low energy part of the pulse-height spectrum. The optimum choice of proton energy is thus a matter which requires several factors to be considered. For much work, 2–4 MeV is required as an appropriate range for effective application of the method.

Although work of this type has generally favoured the use of proton beams, α-particles have also been used. In order to achieve comparable velocities, energies four times greater are needed. This increases the likelihood of nuclear reactions occuring in light elements (notwithstanding the fact that the Coloumb

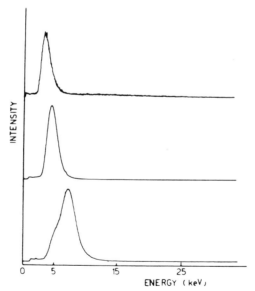

Fig. 7.7   Bremsstrahlung spectra from graphite for proton beam energies of 1.8 MeV (top), 3 MeV (middle) and 4 MeV (bottom). The progressive displacement towards higher energies as the proton energy rises is clearly demonstrated (Berti *et al.* 1977)

barrier is twice as high for α-particles as for protons), and this would contribute to an increased background. Furthermore, the higher particle energy leads to an increased heat dissipation in a thick target, imposing tighter limits on the current which may be used on biological specimens.

Radioactive α-emitters may be made use of to excite characteristic radiation in the samples for analysis. A very 'close' geometry is favoured for this purpose, often with an annular source, using a small sample placed one or two cm away from the source. The system is thus very compact. Exposures of one or two hours may be necessary to obtain adequate counting statistics.

Even heavier particles have also been used, and the production cross-section for x-rays then varies in a somewhat complex manner with the atomic number of the projectile. Broadly speaking, the cross-section passes through a maximum if there is an electronic energy level in the projectile which is close in value to the binding energy of the appropriate electrons in the target atoms. It is therefore possible to achieve some degree of selectivity in analytical procedures by suitable choice of projectile. The potential of heavy-ion induced x-ray emission analysis has by no means been fully explored, although a valuable discussion of the problems involved, together with experimental data, has been given by Cross *et al.* (1977).

7.2 ANALYSIS BY RUTHERFORD BACKSCATTERING

At the energies under discussion, the impact parameter of collisions will usually be many nuclear radii. Scattering angles are therefore usually small. However, about 1 in 10^5 of the incident particles will undergo scattering through a large angle. In these circumstances the nucleus will be 'knocked-on', with measureable energy, the α-particle energy will change, and the change of energy can be made use of in analysis.

By considering a head-on (zero impact parameter) collision, and conserving energy and momentum, it is readily established that

$$\frac{v'}{v} = \frac{1 - M_{proj}/M_{nucl}}{1 + M_{proj}/M_{nucl}}, \tag{7.4}$$

where v and v' are respectively the incident and backscattered velocities of the projectile, and M_{proj} and M_{nucl} are respectively the masses of projectile and struck nucleus. The greatest change of velocity is observed for light elements, which is just the Z-region where x-ray emission analysis is difficult or impossible because of the low fluorescence yield of light elements and the low penetrability of the soft characteristic radiation produced. For heavier elements the change in energy is less, and in such circumstances (7.4) may be seen to approach

$$\frac{v'}{v} = 1 - 2\frac{M_{proj}}{M_{nucl}}. \tag{7.5}$$

Protons which are incident on a heavy element of $Z = 80$ or more will experience less than 1% change in energy, although the possibility of detection is improved somewhat by the Z^2 (target) dependence of the Rutherford scattering cross-section.

Clearly the energy shift of the projectile may be increased by using heavier charged particles, and accordingly beams of α-particles are preferred to protons for this technique. The z^2 (projectile) dependence of the Rutherford cross-section is then an added advantage.

For the detection of the scattered α-particles a small surface-barrier detector is normally used, at an angle of $120°$–$150°$ to the forward beam. At a well-defined angle, and for a thin target, the scattered particles are monoenergetic, but if the target has a finite thickness, or if it consists of a thin surface layer deposited on a substrate of another material, the particles will suffer varying amounts of energy-loss on their way through the surface layer. The spectrum of scattered particles will exhibit a sharp upper limit calculated from (7.4), but will have an extension to lower energies. The width of the broadened peak is therefore a function of layer thickness and can be used for the determination of the thickness and composition of surface deposits such as oxide layers.

This technique has also been used for the study of diffusion profiles at or near the surface of solid materials, and also for the study of ion-implanted layers, where a knowledge of the depth concentration profile may be required.

In the biological field, the potential of Rutherford scattering has been demonstrated by Colautti *et al.* (1976), who have examined the problems of the preparation of thin uniform samples, and who have obtained spectra from samples of rat liver on an aluminium formvar backing. This is illustrated in Fig. 7.8. The

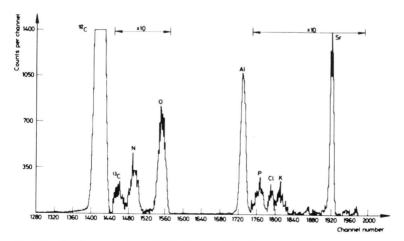

Fig. 7.8   Elastic scattering of 6 MeV α-particles from a rat liver sample on an aluminium formvar backing. Total charge 1030 μC. The internal standard was strontium (3400 ppm), and the spectrum was obtained using a current of 15 nA
(Colautti *et al.* 1976)

principal elements are clearly displayed (the strontium being an added internal standard) and the light elements oxygen, nitrogen and carbon are measurable with ease and could be used as a basis for quantitative determination. Clearly the Rutherford scattering technique forms a potentially useful complement to proton-induced x-ray methods, which are normally confined to $Z > 10$.

It is interesting that the two stable isotopes of carbon are well separated in the spectrum illustrated in Fig. 7.8 (the natural abundance of ^{13}C is 1%), which is a further feature of Rutherford scattering which may be of value in biological applications.

7.3 ANALYSIS BY NUCLEAR REACTIONS

The energies discussed so far in this chapter have been insufficient to cause the charged particles to enter the nucleus, or to come within range of nuclear forces, but at somewhat higher energies nuclear reactions do become possible. A whole range of analytical possibilities is opened up. Using charged-particle induced reactions, we may, in principle at least, make use of (a) promptly-emitted particle spectra; (b) promptly-emitted γ-radiation; (c) delayed particles (that is from induced radioactivity) and (d) delayed γ-ray spectra, from the same cause. We now discuss briefly each of these four situations in turn.

Promptly-emitted particle spectra can be examined by means of a surface barrier detector for protons or α-particles, (neutron spectra may be studied but have not so far been used for analytical work). Charged-particle spectra may ensue from reactions such as (p,α), (α,p), (d,p), on many elements and each reaction yields its own characteristic particle spectrum in which the energies are determined by the incident charged-particle energy, the Q value of the reaction, and the excited state of the product nucleus or intermediate (compound) nucleus. The study of nuclear energy levels by spectroscopy of the reaction products has, in fact, been one of the central preoccupations of experimental nuclear physics for many years. In the present context we are referring, in effect, to the use of these techniques in reverse, for the analysis of samples of material in which quantitative information on, for example, the thickness or the depth distribution of nuclides of known nuclear properties is sought.

The method of 'prompt radiation analysis' has been applied to the study of the thickness of surface layers on various substrates. For example, Wolicki and Knudson (1967) have obtained quantitative information on the thickness of sulphur films using the $^{32}S(d,p)^{33}S$ reaction. Thin oxide layers have been studied using the reactions $^{16}O(d,p)^{17}O$ and $^{18}O(p,\alpha)^{15}N$. Biological applications have been reported by Amsel, for the determination of isotopic composition in biological tissue. In this work, a tantalum electrode was introduced into the tissue and a thin layer of oxygen deposited by the method of anodic oxidation. The isotopic composition of the oxide layer could then be determined by charged-particle bombardment. The technique of obtaining the oxide layer is thus separated from the subsequent charged-particle bombardment, and an interesting feature of the work is that it was found possible to carry out *in vivo* investigations on oxygen metabolism in the rat brain, using ^{18}O as a (stable) isotopic tracer.

A further example illustrates the ease with which isotopic composition may be studied. Fig. 7.9 illustrates a spectrum obtained from the (d,p) reaction on pure graphite. The contribution from ^{13}C is readily seen and could be made the basis of studies of isotopic fractionation in chemical or biological systems.

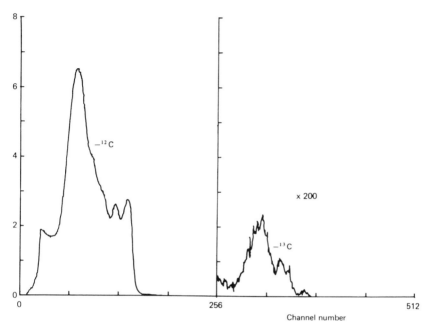

Fig. 7.9 Proton spectrum from the (d,p) reaction on pure graphite (Earwaker and Parvaiz Ali, unpublished)

The γ-radiation emitted during nuclear reactions can be used for analytical purposes, and in this connection we may note that many nuclear reactions are resonant in nature. Proton capture in, for example, ^{27}Al or ^{19}F shows very strong resonances, only a few keV in width, and reactions such as the ^{19}F(p,γ)^{16}O have been used by several workers to study the depth distribution of elements in surface layers. The depth distribution of fluorine in tooth enamel has been studied using this reaction, and also the depth profile of fluorine in metallic samples. Depth resolutions of 20–100 nm have been reported, and can in some circumstances be improved upon.

The remaining methods refer to the observations of induced radioactivity following charged-particle bombardment. The samples can then of course be removed from the target chamber and can be investigated by spectroscopic methods appropriate to the radionuclides formed in the bombardment. Alternatively, autoradiographic methods may be employed to show the spatial distribution of the reaction products. When used for biological work, charged-particle radioactivation techniques are best confined to material which is predominantly mineral in content, because of the degradation which would occur in soft tissue in the beam. Fig.7.10 illustrates autoradiography of a section through a 'staghorn-shaped' urinary calculus, in which the density variations are due mainly to changes in calcium content as the stone developed. The activities induced in the specimen decay with differeing half-lives, and so by taking autoradiographs at different times after the end of bombardment, more than one element can be investigated. A further development has been the use of solid-state nuclear track detectors, to show the distribution of induced α-emitting radioactivity in a sample following charged-particle bombardment. These detectors consist of plastic foils which undergo radiation damage when α-particles are slowed down in them. These trails of damage can be 'revealed' by subsequent etching, and the areal density of the tracks (which may be counted with an optical microscope) enables the spatial distribution of the α-emitter to be determined. The distribution of lead in teeth, using ^{3}He bombardment to yield α-emitting isotopes of polonium has been studied by Al-Niami et al. (1980), and the environmental implications of these observations, particularly in relation to abnormally high concentrations, are also discussed by these authors.

As a final example we look briefly at the photonuclear reactions which take place when matter is irradiated with γ-radiation. We have already noted the occurrence of these reactions, in our discussion of γ-ray interactions in section 1.12.

In general, γ-ray energies in excess of about 8 MeV are required, and for analytical purposes the intense beams of bremsstrahlung obtainable from linear accelerators and betatrons are used. The (γ,n), (γ,p) and (γ,α) reactions are among those found useful for this type of work. Cross-sections tend to be small for these reactions. For example, the cross-section for the ^{197}Au$(\gamma,n)^{196}$Au reaction is only 550 mb compared with 99 b for the ^{197}Au$(n,\gamma)^{198}$Au reaction using thermal neutrons. However, for the study of biological material, photon activation has certain advantages over neutron activation. If analysis of carbon, nitrogen or oxygen is needed, the neutron capture reactions cannot be used because stable products ensue. With photon activation, radioactive products ^{11}C, ^{13}N, ^{15}O readily identifiable by their half-lives (of 20 min, 10 min and 2 min respectively) are produced. Furthermore, neutron activation analysis is sometimes inconvenienced by the preponderance of ^{24}Na activity produced by neutron capture in sodium, and radiochemical separation after irradiation may be required to remove this activity. In the case of photon activation analysis, a small yield of ^{22}Na is produced by the (γ,n) reaction which is not inconvenient.

For effective application of the method, several grams of material are needed, and so the method is very suitable for studies of environmental material such as

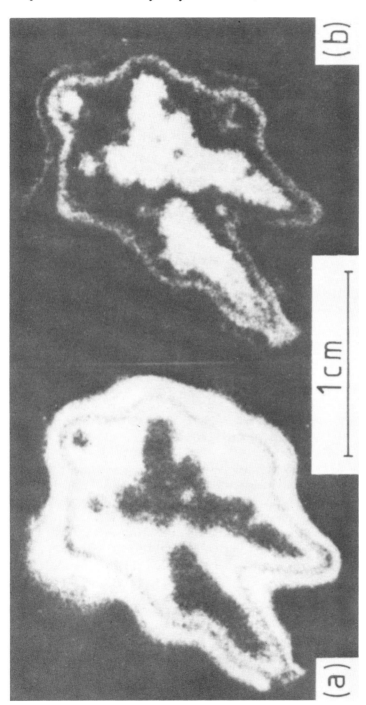

Fig. 7.10 Autoradiography of a section through a urinary stone, following charged-particle bombardment. (a) Carbon; (b) Calcium (McConville, 1980)

soil samples, water, grass or vegetable matter. Detailed investigations have been reported, by Jervis *et al.* (1977), of measurements carried out on hair samples from population exposed to environmental pollutants. Chattopadhyay and Jervis (1974) have reported a study of the measurement of several trace and minor elements in soil samples.

7.4 MUONS AND PIONS IN RADIOBIOLOGY AND MEDICAL PHYSICS

In recent years much interest has been shown in the potential value of less familiar particles in medical and biological science. In this final section we look briefly at the possible applications of muons and pions (μ- and π-mesons) in these fields. Although these particles have long been familiar to nuclear physicists, it is only recently that their potential for applied research has been appreciated.

Pions are particles with a mass equal to approximately 273 electron masses, and spin zero. They are unstable, the π^+ and π^- having life times of 2.6×10^{-8} sec, and the π^0 0.73×10^{-16} sec. The muons (μ^+ and μ^-) have a mass of 207 electron masses, and spin ½. Their lifetime is 2.2×10^{-6} sec. We are here interested in the π^- and μ^- mesons because they can readily be captured by atoms forming orbits which are closely analogous to electronic orbits. This leads to the emission of 'mesic *x*-rays', as the bound meson undergoes transitions to states of successively lower energy, and, in the case of the pion, to capture by the nucleus. We shall see the significance of these two processes shortly. Pions are present in the cosmic radiation, resulting from the interaction of high energy protons in the primary cosmic radiation with atoms in the upper atmosphere. The pions decay to muons, and at sea-level the muons, together with electrons produced by muon decay, form the main component. In the laboratory, pions are produced by proton bombardment of light nuclei, and, although the threshold for pion production is as low as 180 MeV, proton beams of 500 MeV or greater are used, to produce useful yields.

Pions are slowed down in matter by processes closely analagous to the slowing down of fast electrons, and the Bethe–Bloch expression (for example (1.2)) has been found to be valid for calculations of π^- energy-loss. They have a relatively low LET until they approach the end of their range, when the LET rises in accordance with the Bragg curve (which is illustrated, for α-particles, in Fig. 1.2). The penetration of energetic pions (> 60 MeV) is 10–15 cm, in water or in biological tissue, and this, combined with the rising LET towards the end of the range, means that pion beams have a depth dose distribution which is clearly superior to other radiations, in that they alone are able to deliver a radiation dose matching the likely position and extent of a deep-seated tumour, without delivering too high a dose to the overlying tissue. The range can, of course, be adjusted by suitable choice of pion energy, or by the interposition of slowing-down material in the beam.

A further important feature of the negative pions is that they are captured by atoms, cascading through orbits of successively smaller radii until they are captured by nuclei. This process occurs much more rapidly than the natural decay process (which is normally $\pi^- \to \mu^- + \nu$), and nuclear capture results in the production of a variety of light fragments ('star' formation) such as p, ^{3}He, T, and α-particles. These deposit their energy locally with a high LET, and therefore may be expected to possess some of the advantages of high LET radiations discussed in Chapter 6, namely a high relative biological efficiency and a reduced oxygen enhancement ratio, with their attendant potential advantages for the radiotherapy of anoxic tumours. The depth distribution of energy from 95 MeV π^- mesons is illustrated in Fig. 7.11, which shows the contribution from various mechanisms. Star formation occurs at the point of capture, which is at a depth slightly greater than the Bragg peak.

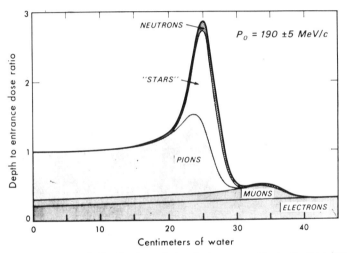

Fig. 7.11   Calculated distribution of absorbed energy with depth for a beam of 95 MeV π^--mesons (Curtis and Raju, 1968)

Radiobiological studies have been carried out using pion beams, for example by Loughman *et al.* (1968). In their investigation, an *in vivo* mammalian cell system was investigated for the induction of polyploidy (that is the production of cell nuclei with abnormally large numbers of chromosomes), by irradiation with 90 MeV negative pions. From their observations, they were able to deduce an RBE of 1 in the flat ('plateau') region of the Bragg curve, rising to 2.15 in the peak. After allowing for the effect of contaminants in the beam (muons and electrons, for which an RBE of 1 was assumed) the RBE for pion effects was found to be 2.37, and for 'star' effects, 3.64. Studies by other investigators have established a diminished oxygen effect (see for example Raju *et al.* 1978). The particular form of the depth dose distribution combined with the delivery of a dose at high LET thus provides a potentially important tool for radiobiological studies and, ultimately, for radiotherapy.

After the negative pion becomes bound by an atom it cascades to successively lower orbits until nuclear capture occurs. During the atomic transitions, energy is radiated in the form of electromagnetic radiation, or as Auger electrons. The electromagnetic radiation is closely analogous to the characteristic x-rays emitted from singly ionized atoms, in that its energy varies smoothly from element to element, and so the term **mesic x-rays** has become established.

In fact the theory of the bound states of negative mesons can be developed along the same lines as for electrons. The binding energies may be written as

$$E_x = \frac{\tfrac{1}{2}mc^2(\alpha Z)^2}{n_x^2} \tag{7.6}$$

where m is now the mass of the meson, and n_x the principal quantum number ($n_x = 1, 2, 3 \ldots$ for the K, L, M ... shells). The orbit radius is given by

$$x = 4\pi\epsilon_0 \cdot \frac{1}{Z} \frac{\hbar^2}{me^2} n_x^2 . \tag{7.7}$$

In the case of π^- mesons, then, we see that the binding energies are **higher** than for electrons, by a factor equal to the ratio of the pion to the electron mass. The orbit radii are **reduced** by this factor, so that the radii of the shells responsible for the main mesic x-ray transitions lie completely inside the electron shells. Screening effects are therefore absent. We may note further that the π-meson may occupy any orbit, and is not restricted by the presence of electrons in the system (the Pauli exclusion principle applies only to **identical** particles). The transitions are thus those pertaining to a hydrogenic atom, giving rise to several series of lines which are closely analogous to the spectra observed in the ultra violet and visible regions. Mesic x-rays in fact can be recognised as forming Lyman and Balmer series, as in the case of optical spectra.

These mesic x-rays are observable when mesons are stopped in matter, and it has been proposed that they could be made the basis of an elemental identification technique. Electronic x-rays have a rather low penetration in matter, and although this does not prevent observations of fluorescent x-rays from elements of moderately high Z in superficial tissues (notably the measurement of iodine concentration in the thyroid) by the use of an external γ-source for excitation, measurements of low Z elements are difficult because of the low photon energies, and the low fluorescence yields, associated with light elements. By contrast, π-mesic x-rays have photon energies typically in excess of 100 keV, which suffer relatively little self-absorption during their outward travel through the overlying tissue, and which can readily be detected by a scintillation counter or Ge(Li) detector. It should be noted, however, that the pion is absorbed into the nucleus with rather high probability, and, because the shell radius varies as Z^{-1}, the probability increases with increasing Z. In fact the K spectrum is observed only for elements with $Z < 9$ and the L spectrum for $Z < 30$. However, other negatively charged mesons can also give rise to x-rays and detailed studies have been carried out using the μ-meson. Muonic x-rays are somewhat lower in energy than pionic x-rays, which follows from the smaller mass of the muon, but the muons interact only weakly with atomic nuclei and so the K and L x-rays are observable throughout the whole range of the elements.

If the orbit radius be calculated for a muonic atom in its ground state (using (7.7)) it is seen that, for atoms of moderately high atomic number, it is substantially less than the nuclear radius. The effective Z is now less than the actual atomic number, because most of the nuclear charge lies **outside** the muonic orbit. The binding energies, and hence the x-ray photon energies are substantially reduced as a consequence of this. However their energies have been determined experimentally for a number of elements and have been tabulated by, for example, Wu and Wilets (1969).

To demonstrate the potential of mesic x-rays for elemental analysis, Taylor, Coulson and Philips (1973) have observed muonic x-rays from biological material *in vitro* (in a bovine femur) and identified calcium and phosphorus in the muonic x-ray spectra (K_α energies of 784 and 457 keV respectively). It was also demonstrated that useful data could be obtained at radiation doses which were acceptably small for human *in vivo* work. Spectra of pionic x-rays obtained from soft biological tissue have recently been published by Jackson (1981) showing lines of the Balmer series from carbon and oxygen.

Clearly, new fields have been opened up by the studies described in this section. Topics which hitherto may have been regarded as the province of the 'pure' physicist are now clearly relevant to the applied sciences. There is a real need to keep abreast of these newer fields, if we are to be aware of the directions in which the applications of nuclear physics to medical and biological problems might move in the future.

FURTHER READING

Ziegler, J. F. (ed.) (1975) *New uses of ion accelerators* Plenum Press

REFERENCES

Al-Niami, T., Edmonds, M. I. and Fremlin, J. H. (1980) *Phys. Med. Biol.*, **25**, 719

Amsel, G. (1973) *J. Radioanal. Chem.*, **17**, 15

Berti, M., Buso, G., Colautti, P., Moschini, G., Stievano, B. M. and Tregnaghi, C. (1977) *Anal. Chem.*, **49**, 1313

Chattopadhyay, A. and Jervis, R. E. (1974) *Anal. Chem.*, **46**, 1630

Colautti, P., Moschini, G. and Stievano, B. M. (1976) *J. Radioanal. Chem.*, **34**, 171

Cross, J. B., Zeisler, R. and Schweikert, E. A. (1977) *Nucl. Instr. and Meth.*, 142, 111

Curtis, S. B. and Raju, M. R. (1968) *Radiation Res.*, 34, 239

Dyson, N. A. (1975) *Phys. Med. Biol.*, 20, 1

Dyson, N. A., Simpson, A. E. and Dabek, J. T. (1978) *J. Radioanal. Chem.*, 46, 309

Garcia, J. D. (1970) *Phys. Rev.*, A1, 1402

Garcia, J. D., Fortner, R. J. and Kavanagh, T. M. (1973) *Revs. Mod. Phys.*, 45, 111

Huda, W. and Bewley, D. K. (1979) *Phys. Med. Biol.*, 24, 711

Hunt, A. H., Parr, R. M., Taylor, D. M. and Trott, N. G. (1963) *Brit. Med. J.*, II, 1498

Jackson, D. F. (1981) *Phys. Bull.*, 32, 48

Jervis, R. E., Tienfenbach, B. and Chattopadhyay, A. (1977) *J. Radioanal. Chem.*, 37, 751

Kemp, K., Palmgren Jensen, F., Tscherning Moller, J. and Gyrd-Hansen, N. (1975) *Phys. Med. Biol.*, 20, 834

Loughman, W. D., Feda, J. M., Raju, M. R. and Winchell, H. S. (1968) *Radiation Res.*, 34, 56

McConville, B. E. (1980) *Brit. J. Urol.*, 52, 243

Merzbacher, E. and Lewis, H.W. (1958) *Encyclopaedia of Physics* (ed. S. Flugge) 34, Springer-Verlag

Raith, R., Roth, M., Gollner, K., Gonsior, B., Ostermann, H. and Uhlhorn, D. (1977) *Nucl. Instr. Meth.*, 142, 39

Raju, M. R. and 11 collaborators (1978) *Brit. J. Radiol.*, 51, 720 (Parts I-IV)

Taylor, M. C., Coulson, L. and Philips, G. C. (1973) *Radiation Res.*, 54, 335

Ward, T. R. and Dyson, N. A. (1978) *J. Phys. B.*, 11, 2705

Wolicki, E. A. and Knudson, A. R. (1967) *Int. J. Appl. Rad. Isotopes*, 18, 429

Wu, C. S. and Wilets, L. (1969) *Ann. Rev. Nucl. Sci.*, 19, 527

Appendices

A1 THE BETHE-BLOCH EXPRESSION FOR ENERGY-LOSS

The loss of energy from a beam of charged particles occurs as a result of ionization of the slowing-down medium, and also by radiative processes. The ionization process is normally predominant, and finds quantitative expression in the Bethe–Bloch formula. The problem may be analysed classically by examining the trajectory of the incident particle.

Referring to Fig. A1.1, we may apply the conservation laws to establish that

$$v_2 = 2v_1 \frac{M}{M+m} \cos \phi_L \tag{A1.1}$$

where v_1 is the velocity of the incident particle (mass M) before the collision and v_2 is the velocity of the struck particle (mass m) after the collision.

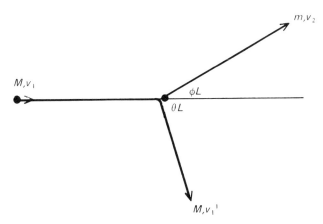

Fig. A1.1 Collision between mass M (in motion) and mass m (initially at rest) in the laboratory system

Fig. A1.1 is in laboratory coordinates. To proceed further we need to examine the system in centre-of-mass coordinates. The collision then appears as in Fig. A1.2. The velocity of the centre of mass relative to the laboratory is given by

$$V = \frac{M}{M+m} v_1 \tag{A1.2}$$

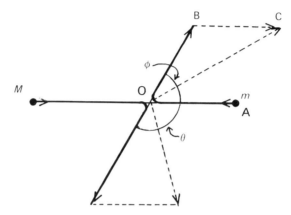

Fig. A1.2   The same collision in centre-of-mass coordinates (BC is the velocity of the centre of mass relative to the laboratory)

Analysis of the system establishes the following:

$$AO = OB, \quad \text{and hence} \quad \phi = 2\phi_L$$

$$\phi = \pi - \theta \quad \text{hence} \quad \phi_L = \frac{\pi}{2} - \frac{\theta}{2}$$

If we denote $\frac{1}{2} mv_2^2$, the energy transferred to the struck particle, by Q, we find that

$$Q = Q_0 \sin^2 \frac{\theta}{2}, \quad \text{where} \tag{A1.3}$$

$$Q_0 = \frac{1}{2} m \left(2v_1 \frac{M}{M+m}\right)^2 \tag{A1.4}$$

The path of the incident charged particle moving under the influence of a central Coulomb force is a hyperbola, and by detailed analysis of its motion may be established the expression

$$p = \frac{b}{2} \cot \frac{\theta}{2}, \quad \text{where} \quad b = \frac{1}{4\pi\epsilon_0} \frac{2zZe^2}{M_0 v_1^2} \tag{A1.5}$$

ze and Ze are the charges on the incident and struck particles respectively ($Z = 1$ for the struck electron), and M_0 is the reduced mass of the 2-particle system,

$$M_0 = \frac{Mm}{m + M} \tag{A1.6}$$

Physically, b is equal to the distance of closest approach between repelling particles in a head-on collision, although this analysis applies both to repelling collisions (as with a beam of electrons) and attractive collisions (for example a beam of α-particles), remembering that the struck particle is an electron in each case. (Fig. A1.3).

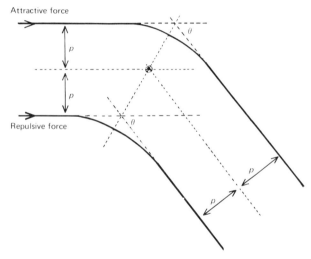

Fig. A1.3 For a given impact parameter (and a given value of b) the angles of deflection are the same irrespective of whether the force is attractive or repulsive

From (A1.3) and (A1.5) it may readily be established that

$$Q = Q_0 \frac{b^2/4}{p^2 + b^2/4} \tag{A1.7}$$

Large impact parameters therefore correspond to small energy transfers.

To obtain dE, the kinetic energy transferred in a distance dx, we need to integrate over all impact parameters

$$dE = \left[\int_{p_{min}}^{p_{max}} QnZ \, 2\pi p \, dp \right] dx,$$

where nZ the number of electrons per unit volume.

If we now make the assumption that b is small compared with p (which is equivalent to the statement that the scattering angle is usually small), we may write

$$Q = Q_0 \frac{b^2}{4p^2}$$

Hence
$$\frac{dE}{dx} = \int_{p_{min}}^{p_{max}} \frac{Q_0 b^2}{4p^2} nZ 2\pi p\, dp$$

$$= \frac{\pi}{2} Q_0 b^2 nZ \ln \frac{p_{max}}{p_{min}} \tag{A1.8}$$

The choice of p_{max} and p_{min} gives rise to some difficulty. It may be supposed that no net energy will be transferred if the time of interaction exceeds the period of the electron orbit. The time of interaction is of order p/v, and the orbit period is of order h/I where I is the ionization potential.

Hence $p_{max} = \dfrac{hv}{I}$

The impact parameter cannot realistically be less than the wavelength of the struck electron as seen by the moving particle, that is

$$p_{min} = \frac{h}{mv}$$

Inserting these limits, and using (A1.4) and (A1.5) for Q_0 and b, we obtain

$$\frac{dE}{dx} = \left(\frac{1}{4\pi\epsilon_0}\right)^2 \frac{4\pi z^2 e^4}{mv^2} nZ \ln \frac{mv^2}{I} \tag{A1.9}$$

This is a valid form of the Bethe–Bloch formula. If, however, it is compared with (1.2) and (1.3) it is seen to differ in three respects. First, the numerical coefficient within the logarithmic term differs by a factor of 2. The effect of this is small, and in any case we have already noted (section 1.3) that different treatments yield somewhat different values for this factor. Secondly, the quantity I must be modified in order to obtain a mean value of all possible excitation potentials as well as the ionization potential, and, in the case of many-electron atoms, all possible ionization potentials. This mean value is expressed as $\bar{J}$ in (1.3) and is discussed there. Thirdly, (1.2) includes some relativistic corrections which are significant for swift particles and which can be derived by a more detailed treatment.

The Bethe-Bloch formula has been found to be of value in a very wide variety of conditions including the slowing-down of positrons, μ- and π-measons and heavy ions.

A2 THE KLEIN-NISHINA FORMULA

The Klein–Nishina formula may be expressed in several different ways, and we here summarise a few important results.

If we consider plane-polarised radiation, and examine only the cases where the scattering plane (that is the plane containing the direction of incidence and the direction of scattered radiation) contains also the electric vector of the incident radiation (Fig. A2.1), the differential collision cross-section for Compton scattering is given by

$$d\sigma = \frac{r_e^2}{2} d\omega \left(\frac{\nu^1}{\nu}\right)^2 \left(\frac{\nu}{\nu^1} + \frac{\nu^1}{\nu} - 2\sin^2\theta\right) \tag{A2.1}$$

where r_e is the classical electron radius (section 1.9), ν and ν^1 are the frequencies of the incident and scattered radiation (related via (1.33), with $E = h\nu$ and $E^1 = h\nu^1$) and θ is the scattering angle.

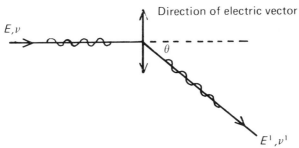

Fig. A2.1 Illustrating Compton scattering when the electric vector of the incident radiation lies in the scattering plane (see text)

When $\nu^1 \rightarrow \nu$, this expression approaches

$$d\sigma = r_e^2 d\omega \cos^2\theta,$$

which is the angular distribution for Thomson scattering of plane polarised radiation (1.42).

$\dfrac{\nu^1}{\nu}$ may be written in the form (from 1.33)

$$\frac{\nu^1}{\nu} = \frac{1}{1 + \alpha(1 - \cos\theta)} \tag{A2.2}$$

As the frequency shift becomes greater (whether because of an increase in α or in θ) the differential cross-section falls below the Thomson value, showing that the angular distribution becomes more peaked in the forward direction. This becomes progressively more marked as the incident photon energy is increased.

A more complete form of (A2.1) is

$$d\sigma = \frac{r_e^2}{2} d\omega \left(\frac{\nu^1}{\nu}\right)^2 \left(\frac{\nu}{\nu^1} + \frac{\nu^1}{\nu} - 2 \sin^2\theta \cos^2\eta\right) \qquad (A2.3)$$

where η is the angle between the plane defined by the direction of incidence and the direction of the electric vector of the incident radiation, and the scattering plane. For unpolarised radiation we require the average value of $\cos^2\eta$, which is $\frac{1}{2}$, leading to

$$d\sigma = \frac{r_e^2}{2} d\omega \left(\frac{\nu^1}{\nu}\right)^2 \left(\frac{\nu}{\nu^1} + \frac{\nu^1}{\nu} - \sin^2\theta\right). \qquad (A2.4)$$

The **intensity** scattered at an angle θ into a solid angle $d\omega$ is given by this expression multiplied by a further factor of ν^1/ν.

The differential cross-section for scattering through an angle θ (A2.4) is illustrated for different incident photon energies in Fig. A2.2.

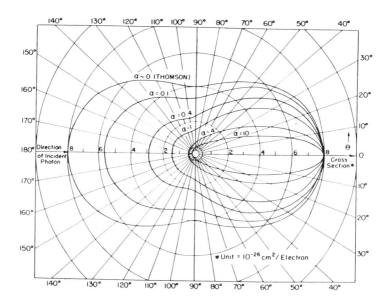

Fig. A2.2 The differential cross-section for Compton scattering of unpolarised radiation, as a function of angle (Davisson and Evans, 1952)

To obtain the total collision cross-section, (A2.4) requires integration over all scattering angles. The result is

$$\sigma = 2\pi r_e^2 \left[\frac{1+\alpha}{\alpha^3} \left\{ \frac{2\alpha(1+\alpha)}{(1+2\alpha)} - \ln(1+2\alpha) \right\} + \frac{\ln(1+2\alpha)}{2\alpha} - \frac{1+3\alpha}{(1+2\alpha)^2} \right].$$

$$(A2.5)$$

This is the function illustrated in Fig. 1.12.

REFERENCE

Davisson, C. M. and Evans, R. D. (1952) *Revs. Mod. Phys.*, **24**, 79

A3 THE SEMI-EMPIRICAL MASS FORMULA

Certain properties of nuclei, particularly those relating to mechanisms of radio-active decay, may be explained on the basis of relatively simple assumptions regarding the forces between nucleons. The assumption is made that a nucleon interacts with all its nearest neighbours and that the nuclear force, or strong interaction, is a short range force, so that interactions between nucleons not in 'contact' may be neglected.

If a nucleus consists of N neutrons and Z protons ($A = N + Z$), the main term in the nuclear mass-energy must be

$$M = NM_n + ZM_p \qquad (A3.1)$$

where M_n and M_p are the masses of the neutron and proton respectively. The **binding energy** must be **subtracted** from this expression to give the net mass-energy, and consists of the following terms:

1. A 'volume' term, expressing the fact that there are A nucleons, each with a binding energy which we denote by an empirically determined constant c_v. That is the volume term is given by

$$B_v = c_v A.$$

2. A 'surface energy term', which takes account of the fact that certain nucleons are at the nuclear surface and are therefore bound less strongly. The nuclear volume is proportional to A, the nuclear radius to $A^{1/3}$, and the nuclear surface area to $A^{2/3}$. Therefore the surface term is given by

$$B_s = -c_s A^{2/3}.$$

3. A 'coulomb term', expressing the coulomb repulsion between the protons.
From electrostatistics this is given by

$$-\frac{1}{4\pi\epsilon_0}\frac{\frac{3}{5}(Ze)^2}{R}$$

where R is the nuclear radius.

4. An 'asymmetry' term: The binding energy of a nucleus is (if coulomb forces
are absent) minimal if there are equal numbers of protons and neutrons. If there
is an excess of neutrons over protons they are, as it were, forced into higher
energy level and are thereby prevented from the complete binding implied by
the saturation of nuclear forces. If the neutron excess is given by n, and the
average spacing between nuclear levels is ϵ, the reduction of binding energy is
given by

$$\epsilon[n + (n - 1) + (n - 2) \ldots\ldots 2 + 1]$$

$$\approx \frac{\epsilon n^2}{2} = \frac{\epsilon}{2}(N - Z)^2.$$

This is usually written as $\quad + \dfrac{c_a(N - Z)^2}{A}$.

5. A 'pairing' term.
  If there are **even** numbers of neutrons and protons, the binding is **increased**
by an amount which may be written as $+\Delta_i$. If the number of neutrons and
protons are each **odd**, the binding is **decreased** by this amount. The pairing term
is arbitrarily zero if there is an odd number of neutrons and an even number of
protons, or vice versa.
  We therefore have, in the binding energy, a term δ, which is equal to

$\quad +\Delta$ for even–even nuclei
$\quad -\Delta$ for odd–odd nuclei
$\quad\;\; 0$ for odd–even (that is odd A) nuclei.

Remembering that these five binding energy terms must be subtracted from the
mass terms in (A2.1) we may write

$$M = NM_n + ZM_p$$

$$-\frac{1}{c^2}[c_v A - c_s A^{2/3} - \frac{1}{4\pi\epsilon_0}\frac{3}{5}\frac{Z^2 e^2}{R} + c_a\frac{(N-Z)^2}{A} + \delta] \quad (A3.2)$$

which is the semi-empirical mass formula.

A4 THE BREIT-WIGNER FORMULA

In order to explain the resonant nature of the capture of slow neutrons, consider an expression of the form

$$\sigma \propto \frac{\text{const}}{(E - E_0)^2 + \Gamma^2/4} \tag{A4.1}$$

where E is the neutron energy and E_0 the energy at which resonance occurs. This expression was originally used (by Breit and Wigner) based on analogy with the resonant absorption and scattering of light, and may readily be related to resonant processes in other branches of physics. Γ here represents the width of the resonance, in that the cross-section given by (A4.1) will fall to one half of its peak value when $E - E_0 = \Gamma/2$.

The maximum value for the interaction cross-section between an incident particle and a nucleus may be expected to be of the order of πR^2, where R is the nuclear radius (see for example the remarks in section 2.3 on compound nucleus formation). However, in the case of slow neutrons, the effective radius of interaction must be of order $\lambdabar$ where $\lambdabar$ is the reduced de Broglie wavelength ($\lambda = h/p = 2\pi\lambdabar$). The peak cross-section for a neutron entering a nucleus is therefore more likely to be given by

$$\sigma = \pi(\lambdabar + R)^2, \quad \text{or, if} \quad \lambdabar \gg R,$$

$$\pi\lambdabar^2.$$

Further considerations establish that the inclusion of elastic scattering gives, for the total interaction cross-section at the peak

$$\sigma = 4\pi\lambdabar^2. \tag{A4.2}$$

The constant of proportionality in (A4.1) must therefore be given by $\pi\lambdabar^2\Gamma^2$. Hence we may write, from (A4.1),

$$\sigma = \pi\lambdabar^2 \frac{\Gamma^2}{(E - E_0)^2 + \tfrac{1}{4}\Gamma^2} \tag{A4.3}$$

which establishes the constant of proportionality.

For the specific process of de-excitation by the emission of γ-radiation, the cross-section must be multiplied by a factor Γ_γ/Γ where Γ_γ is the partial width for the radiative process, giving

$$\sigma = \pi\lambdabar^2 \frac{\Gamma\Gamma_\gamma}{(E - E_0)^2 + \tfrac{1}{4}\Gamma^2} \tag{A4.4}$$

which is the Breit–Wigner formula for radiative capture of a neutron by a nucleus of zero angular momentum.

At very low neutron energies such that E is well below the lowest resonant energy $(E \ll E_0)$, the denominator of (A4.4) approaches a constant value and

$$\sigma \propto \lambda^2 \Gamma.$$

The slow neutron width Γ is related to the velocity of the neutron, being in fact proportional to it. This may be seen by noting that, if τ is the interaction time of the slow neutron, we may write

$$\Gamma \tau \sim \hbar, \quad \text{hence} \quad \Gamma \propto v.\dagger$$

Hence $\qquad \sigma \propto \lambda^2 v, \quad \text{or} \quad \left(\frac{\hbar}{m v}\right)^2 v,$ $\qquad\qquad\qquad$ (A4.5)

$$\propto \frac{1}{v},$$

establishing the 1/v law for the variation of the (n, γ) reaction cross-section with energy, upon which the resonances are superimposed.

A5 RADIOACTIVE TRANSFORMATIONS – GROWTH AND DECAY

The study of natural radioactivity revealed the existence of radioactive decay chains, in which each radioactive decay process produced a daughter product which was itself radioactive, the chain eventually terminating with a stable isotope of lead or bismuth. Equations to describe the growth and decay of the intermediate members of a chain were set up at an early stage in the study of radioactivity and have been described by many authors. We confine ourselves to the relatively simple situation where the decay chain consists of only three members:

$$A \rightarrow B \rightarrow \underline{C} \quad \text{(stable).}$$

† A more formal approach examines the motion of a free particle, noting that the probability of interaction is proportional to the density of states available to it, in a momentum interval dp. Detailed exposition of this approach would carry us beyond the scope of this book, but if we note that the volume of momentum space accessible to it is given by $4\pi p^2 \, dp$, we may write for the number of available states, which will equal the accessible volume of momentum space in units of h^3,

$$dn = \frac{4\pi p^2 \, dp}{h^3}, \quad \text{and the state density is given by}$$

$$\frac{dn}{dE} = \frac{4\pi p^2}{h^3} \frac{dp}{dE} = \frac{4\pi}{h^3} Mp, \quad \text{which is proportional to v.}$$

If N_a, N_b are the numbers of atom of A and B present at time t, we can write

$$\frac{dN_a}{dt} = -\lambda_a N_a \qquad\qquad (A5.1a)$$

$$\frac{dN_b}{dt} = \lambda_a N_a - \lambda_b N_b \qquad\qquad (A5.1b)$$

A commonly-occurring situation is when there are no atoms of type B present at $t = 0$. So, putting $N_a = N_0$ and $N_b = 0$ at $t = 0$, the following solutions of these equations may be obtained:

$$N_a = N_0 e^{-\lambda_a t} \qquad\qquad (A5.2a)$$

$$N_b = \frac{\lambda_a}{\lambda_b - \lambda_a} N_0 (e^{-\lambda_a t} - e^{-\lambda_b t}) \qquad\qquad (A5.2b)$$

The activities of A_a and A_b are given by $\lambda_a N_a$ and $\lambda_b N_b$ respectively.
    For small values of t, (A5.2b) reduces to

$$N_b = \lambda_a N_0 t, \quad \text{and hence}$$

$$A_b = \lambda_b \lambda_a N_0 t.$$

We see that the daughter activity at first rises linearly with time. Inspection of (A5.2b) shows that the number of atoms (and hence the activity) of the daughter product passes through a maximum and then falls again. It is also apparent that at the time of maximum daughter activity, the activities of parent and daughter are equal. We can distinguish three cases:

1.   The daughter nuclide is shorter-lived than the parent ($\lambda_b > \lambda_a$)

$$\frac{A_b}{A_a} = \frac{\lambda_b}{\lambda_b - \lambda_a} (1 - e^{-(\lambda_b - \lambda_a)t}) \qquad\qquad (A5.3)$$

At long times, therefore

$$\frac{A_b}{A_a} \rightarrow \frac{\lambda_b}{\lambda_b - \lambda_a}, \qquad\qquad (A5.4)$$

and the daughter decays with the half-life of the parent. This situation is known as **transient equilibrium**, and is illustrated in Fig. A5.1. We have met practical examples of this situation in section 2.8.5 in connection with the use of a 'generator' to produce in the laboratory a radioisotope with a half-life which would otherwise be too short for processing and transportation:

$$^{132}\text{Te} \xrightarrow{78\text{h}} {}^{132}\text{I} \xrightarrow{2.6\text{h}} {}^{132}\underline{\text{Xe}} \quad (\text{stable})$$

and (making some simplification of the transformation in the interest of clarity)

$$^{99}\text{Mo} \xrightarrow{67\text{h}} {}^{99\text{m}}\text{Tc} \xrightarrow{6\text{h}} \underset{\cdots}{{}^{99}\underline{\text{Tc}}} \quad (\text{very long half-life}).$$

Fig. A5.1 illustrates these two cases. From equation (A5.4), putting in appropriate values for λ_a and λ_b, we see that the ratio of equilibrium activities would be 1.003 and 1.098 for the $^{132}\text{Te}/^{132}\text{I}$ and $^{99}\text{Mo}/^{99\text{m}}\text{Tc}$ systems respectively.

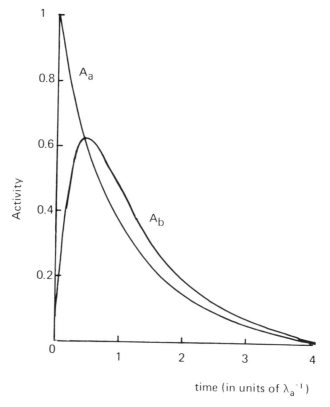

Fig. A5.1 Transient equilibrium between radioactive parent and daughter (see text) for the case when $\lambda_b = 4\lambda_a$

2.   If the disparity of half-lives is very great ($\lambda_b \gg \lambda_a$).

In this case $\dfrac{A_b}{A_a} \to 1,$

and the daughter activity remains equal to the parent activity after equilibrium has been reached. This is known as **secular equilibrium**. An example of this is the growth of the ^{137m}Ba metastable state from ^{137}Cs, which then decays with the ^{137}Cs half-life emitting the 662 keV γ-radiation invariably attributed to ^{137}Cs. Many examples of secular equilibrium are to be found in the natural radioactive series or in the decay chains of fission products.

3.   The daughter is longer-lived than the parent.

(A5.3) shows that the ratio of activities of daughter and parent increases continuously with time, and no equilibrium exists (Fig. A5.2).

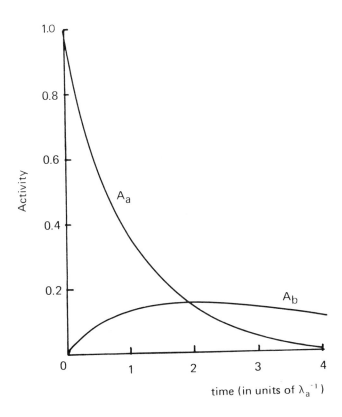

Fig. A5.2 Activities of radioactive parent and daughter when $\lambda_b = \frac{1}{4}\lambda_a$

List of Symbols

This listing shows the physical quantity represented by each symbol, and the location (usually a numbered equation) where the symbol first occurs with the stated meaning.

b	collision distance	(1.18)
M_0	reduced mass	Sec. 1.6
θ_m	angle of scattering in centre-of-mass coordinates	(1.20)
δ	scattering angle	Fig. 1.5(b)
N	number of photons in primary beam	(1.26)
σ	removal cross-section	(1.26)
E_γ, E	photon energy	Sec. 1.8; (1.27)
α, β	constants in equation	(1.27)
G, x	quantities in stationary wave functions	(1.28)
n	principal quantum number	(1.28)
a_H	Bohr hydrogen radius	(1.28)
p	momentum	(1.29a)
E'	energy of scattered photon	(1.29a)
θ	scattering angle of photon	(1.29a)
ϕ	scattering angle of electron	(1.29b)
U	total mass-energy	Sec. 1.9
T	kinetic energy	(1.30a)
λ, λ'	wavelength of incident and scattered radiation	(1.34)
r_e	classical electron radius	footnote, Sec. 1.9
μ_0	permeability of free space	footnote, Sec. 1.9
α	ratio of photon energy to electron rest energy, E_γ/mc^2	(1.35)
W	energy flux in an electromagnetic wave	(1.36)
ω	solid angle	(1.37b)
$E_\mathrm{i}, E_\mathrm{s}$	electron field strength in incident and scattered electromagnetic waves	(1.39)
r	distance from an electromagnetic radiator	(1.39)
τ_m	mean-life of a transition	(1.46)
Γ	width of a nuclear level	(1.46)
p_1, p_2, p_3	probabilities per unit time	Sec. 1.12
g	statistical factor	(1.48)
$I_\mathrm{g}, I_\mathrm{e}$	spins of nuclear ground and excited states	(1.48)
$\lambdabar$	reduced wavelength, $\lambda/2\pi$	Sec. 1.12
Γ_γ	*radiative* width of a nuclear level	(2.2)
a	number of target atoms per unit volume	(2.3)
g	target thickness	(2.3)
σ, σ'	reaction cross-section	(2.3)
λ	radioactive decay constant	(2.3)
n	number of radioactive atoms	(2.3)
N	number of incident particles per unit time	(2.3)

U, U_0	number of target atoms	(2.6), (2.8)
Σ	macroscopic cross-section	Sec. 2.7.1
ϕ	particle flux	(2.6)
V	voltage	(3.1)
C	electrical capacity	(3.1)
W	mean energy required to produce an ion-pair	(3.1)
N_{true}, N_{obs}	true and observed counting rates	(3.2)
τ	dead time (paralysis time) in a counting system	(3.2)
N	number of initial ion-pairs	(3.3)
M	gas multiplication (in a counter for 1 initial electron)	(3.3)
$\bar{M}$	mean value of M averaged over N initial electrons	(3.3)
P	final number of ion-pairs	(3.3)
σ_N, etc.	standard deviation in N, etc.	(3.3)
F	Fano factor (see text)	(3.4)
E	stored electrostatic energy	(3.7)
q	charge in an electrostatic system	(3.8)
q'	induced charge in an electrostatic system	(3.10)
T	electron kinetic energy	Sec. 3.5
E	macroscopic energy absorbed in a medium	Sec. 3.5
$_vE_g, {}_vE_s$	energy absorbed per unit volume in gas and in solid, respectively	(3.14)
$_vJ, {}_mJ$	number of ion pairs produced per unit volume or per unit mass respectively	(3.15)
Q	change in atomic mass-energy in radioactive decay	(4.6)
dp, dq	momentum intervals (in β-decay) for electron and neutrino respectively	(4.10)
g	fundamental weak interaction constant	(4.14)
λ_d	radioactive decay constant	Sec. 4.2
P_r	power radiated from an oscillating dipole	(4.17)
ω	angular frequency of radiated electromagnetic energy	(4.17)
I_i, I_f	nuclear spins of initial and final states	Sec. 4.3
α	internal conversion coefficient	Sec. 4.4
ψ	wave function (ψ^2 = probability, electron density)	(4.19)
ω_k	fluorescence yield (in K-shell)	(4.21)
E_f	Fermi energy	(4.22)
ω	solid angle	(4.24)
ϵ	efficiency (of a radiation detector)	Sec. 4.7
w_1, w_2	proportion by weight	(4.28)
D_β	dose-rate (due to β-particles)	(4.31)
ν	"effective" attenuation coefficient for β-particles	(4.31)
Γ	specific γ-emission of a radionuclide	(4.33)
V, V'	volumes of compartments	Sec. 5.2
C, C'	concentration of a radioactive tracer	(5.1)

Q, q	activities (of a radioactive tracer)	(5.2)
x	number of radioactive atoms present	(5.3)
K	turnover rate constant	(5.3)
τ_b, τ_r	biological, radioactive half-life	Sec. 5.3
R	input of radioactive atoms into a compartment per unit time	(5.4)
α	solubility constant for gases in water	(5.19)
E, E'	neutron kinetic energies	(6.1)
k	Boltzmann's constant	(6.3)
T	temperature	(6.3)
α	fine structure constant	(7.1)
E_k	electron K-shell binding energy	(7.3)
E_p	proton kinetic energy	(7.3)
U	excitation ratio	Sec. 7.1
m	meson mass	(7.6)
R	nuclear radius	App. 3, 4

Index